2ND Edition

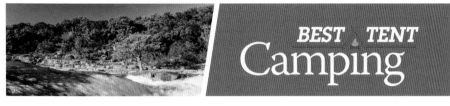

BEST TENT
Camping

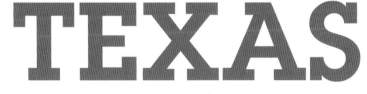

TEXAS

YOUR CAR-CAMPING GUIDE TO SCENIC BEAUTY, THE SOUNDS
OF NATURE, AND AN ESCAPE FROM CIVILIZATION

Best Tent Camping: Texas

Library of Congress Cataloging-in-Publication Data

Names: Withrow, Wendel, author.
Title: Best tent camping Texas : your car-camping guide to scenic beauty, the sounds of nature, and an escape from
   civilization / Wendel Withrow.
Description: 2nd edition. | Birmingham, Alabama : Menasha Ridge Press, 2017. | Includes index. | Revised edition of :
   Best in tent camping Texas : A guide for car campers who hate RVs, concrete slabs, and loud portable stereos /
   Wendel Withrow. c2009.
Identifiers: LCCN 2017031149 | ISBN 9780897324922 (pbk.) | ISBN 9780897324939 (eISBN)
Subjects: LCSH: Camping—Texas—Guidebooks. | Camp sites, facilities, etc.—Texas—Guidebooks. | Texas—Guidebooks.
Classification: LCC GV191.42.T4 W49 2017 | DDC 796.5409764—dc23
LC record available at https://lccn.loc.gov/2017031149

Book design: Jonathan Norberg
Cover design: Scott McGrew
Maps: Steve Jones
Photos: Wendel Withrow and Chase Fountain
Project editor: Holly Cross
Copy editor: Scott Alexander Jones
Proofreader: Laura Franck
Indexer: Ann Cassar

MENASHA RIDGE PRESS
An imprint of AdventureKEEN
2204 First Ave. S., Ste. 102
Birmingham, Alabama 35233
800-443-7227, fax 205-326-1012

Visit menasharidge.com for a complete listing of our books and for ordering information. Contact us at our website, at
facebook.com/menasharidge, or at twitter.com/menasharidge with questions or comments. To find out more about
who we are and what we're doing, visit blog.menasharidge.com.

Front cover: Main: Backcountry campsite in Big Bend National Park; © Fredlyfish4 (via Shutterstock.com).
Inset: Pedernales River and Falls at Pedernales Falls State Park in Texas hill country; © CrackerClips Stock Media
(via Shutterstock.com)

2ND Edition

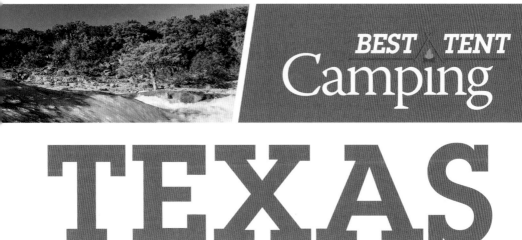

BEST TENT
Camping

TEXAS

YOUR CAR-CAMPING GUIDE TO SCENIC BEAUTY, THE SOUNDS
OF NATURE, AND AN ESCAPE FROM CIVILIZATION

Wendel Withrow

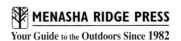

MENASHA RIDGE PRESS
Your Guide to the Outdoors Since 1982

Texas Campground Locator Map

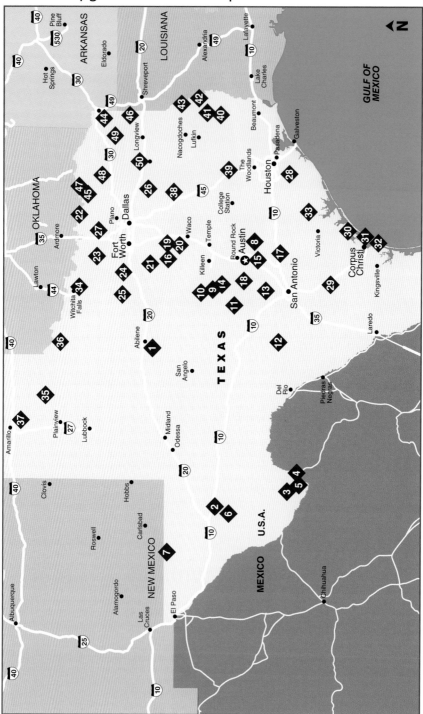

CONTENTS

SOUTH TEXAS AND THE GULF COAST 107

THE TEXAS PANHANDLE, HIGH PLAINS, AND CAPROCK CANYONS 129

DEEP EAST TEXAS AND THE BIG THICKET 145

NORTHEAST TEXAS AND CADDO LAKE AREA 166

Map Legend

N North indicator	← Off-map or pinpoint-indication arrow	Creekside camping area / Campground regular and beach sites

Individual tent sites, RV sites, cabins, huts, and decks

Group site	Austin ✪ — Capital	Waco ● — City or town	**NATIONAL FOREST** **STATE PARK** — Public lands

Main Trail — Hiking, biking, and equestrian

Interstate highways	US highways	State roads	Other roads	Dirt/gravel roads
635 45	183 22	361 22	Park Road 31	

Aircraft runway	Fences	*Colorado River* — River or stream	*Oxbow Lake* — Lake or pond

Amphitheater		Group picnic shelter		Private residence
Baseball		Hiking trail		Recreation hall
Basketball		Historic marker		Recycling bin
Bathhouse		Hitching post		Restroom
Biking trail		Horse campsite		Scenic view
Boat ramp		Horse stables		Screened shelter
Bridge or tunnel		Horse trail		Shelter
Chemical/compost toilet		Horses restricted		Structure or feature
Concession		Horseshoe pit		Summit or lookout
Dining hall		Interpretive trail		Swimming
Dumpster		Laundry		Telephone
Equestrian parking		Maintenance		Trailer dumpsite
Fire hydrant		No-biking trail		Trash
Firewood		No-hiking trail		Volleyball
Fish cleaning		No swimming		Water access
Fishing		Park gift shop		Watering area
Four-wheel drive		Park office		Water/electric sites
Full hookups		Parking		Wheelchair accessible
Gate		Picnic area		Wildlife viewing
Group picnic area		Picnic pavilion		Wind surfing
		Playground		

ACKNOWLEDGMENTS

Thank you for:

The many dedicated and underappreciated state and federal employees who shared their favorite campsites with me so that I can pass them on to you. A special note of appreciation to the technical staff at the Texas Parks & Wildlife Department for the excellent detailed maps of the state park campgrounds, and thanks to Chase Fountain for providing some of the best photography in any guidebook in any state. Chase's work is regularly featured in the *Texas Parks & Wildlife* magazine, which is celebrating its 75th anniversary. Additional thanks go to the magazine's managing editor Russell Roe for his assistance in coordinating the use of Chase Fountain's photos in the second edition.

Molly Merkle, Holly Cross, Karla Linder, Steve Jones, Scott Alexander Jones, and the whole team at Menasha Ridge for their assistance in tackling a project the size of Texas.

Clarke Abbey for permission and the legendary Edward Abbey (1927–1989) for inspiration to share the most important message of all: "One brave deed is worth a thousand books. Sentiment without action is the ruin of the soul."

Lee Stetson (an actor known for his portrayal of Yosemite's John Muir), Doug Peacock (*Grizzly Years: In Search of the American Wilderness*), and Jack Loeffler (*Healing the West: Voices of Culture and Habitat*) for their tireless efforts to defend America's remaining wildlands and pass on the passion of John Muir, Edward Abbey, and countless unsung conservationists to future generations of tent campers and all who love our natural world.

My legal assistant, Donna Ervin, for her technical expertise in preparing the manuscript and never complaining about the extra work.

My research assistants, traveling companions, and trail leaders on the first edition: Philip and Brandon Rothermel, Nick Wood, and Meridynn Barber.

My assistant and outings expert, Liz Wheelan, for her incredible diligence in fact-checking the updates for each park and adding her extensive backcountry travel experience to the whole project.

My parents, Alvin and Lucy Withrow, for passing on to me their love of history and travel, along with the confidence to meet any challenge.

My wife, Ada Marie, for assisting me at many of the campgrounds and being patient at home, where the stacks of park files and background documents seemed to just grow and grow during writing of the first edition and then returning for the second marathon project.

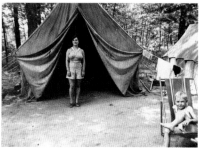

The original tent camper: Lucy Withrow, July 1939

PREFACE

Even under the best of circumstances, any author who takes on the task of writing a camping guidebook for the state of Texas faces a serious challenge. When that same author, in theory older and wiser, solicits the opportunity to write a second edition, then the reader may rightly question whether the author has hiked a few too many miles under that Texas summer sun. An equally good answer is that the first edition has been graciously well received to the extent that it is in its fourth printing, and some of the details needed to be updated. There are also new parks to be added that were temporarily closed by two hurricanes and a few random tornadoes. Large wildfires and the historic floods of 2014–2016 hit other parks listed in the first edition. While every attempt has been made to give the reader the most recent status, be sure to call or check the website of any park you wish to visit.

This second edition offers these new features:

1. Additional recommended reading selections for campers of all interests.
2. More quotes and background in "Voices From the Campfire."
3. A new section titled "Backcountry Adventures" to meet the increased interest and popularity of activities other than traditional hiking and camping.
4. A new section of critical importance titled "Best Local Food and Drink." Of course, the author sampled as many of these non-chain culinary stops as possible, but he also sought input from the locals, who know that real Texas food is often found off the main trail.
5. A new appendix with detailed suggestions for successful day hiking in all types of terrain and conditions.

In choosing the 50 tent campgrounds included in this guide, I took into account not only the criteria explained in the Introduction but also that feeling we all get when we leave the cement jungle for an outdoor adventure and find something special. It may be a spectacular vista, a fiery sunset, a single flower bloom, or even the intoxicating smell of a campfire, but we all sense it as soon as we arrive. As you visit the places described in this simple book, I can only hope you will have the same sense of wonder and receive the gifts of peace that only the natural world can instill in us.

You will also see a list of diverse books (some hard to find) and select quotes from various authors who have come before us and contemplated the eternal struggle between the seemingly unquenchable appetite of modern civilization and the very real need of the individual to leave that world and return to a simpler life, even if just for a short time. This section, titled "Voices from the Campfire and Recommended Reading," relates to one of the most important traditions of tent camping—conversation! Whether the conversation is between childhood friends or new acquaintances, the best type of escape can be found gathering around a crackling wood fire and sharing life's experiences, without a computer screen or cell phone to separate us from our fellow humans. To assist in that escape is the essence of tent camping and the purpose of this book.

—*Wendel Withrow*

BEST
CAMPGROUNDS

BEST FOR BIRD-WATCHING

BEST FOR CANOEING AND KAYAKING

BEST FOR CYCLING AND MOUNTAIN BIKING

BEST FOR EQUESTRIANS

BEST FOR FAMILIES WITH KIDS

BEST FOR FISHING AND BOATING

BEST FOR HIKING

INTRODUCTION

HOW TO USE THIS GUIDEBOOK

THE RATING SYSTEM

As with all books in the Best Tent Camping series, this guidebook's author personally experienced dozens of campgrounds and campsites to select the top 50 locations in this state. Within that universe of 50 sites, the author then ranked each one according to the six categories described below.

Each campground is superlative in its own way. For example, a site may be rated only one star in one category but perhaps five stars in another category. Our rating system allows you to choose your destination based on the attributes that are most important to you. Though these ratings are subjective, they're still excellent guidelines for finding the perfect camping experience for you and your companions.

★★★★★	The site is **ideal** in that category.
★★★★	The site is **exemplary** in that category.
★★★	The site is **very good** in that category.
★★	The site is **above average** in that category.
★	The site is **acceptable** in that category.

INDIVIDUAL RATINGS

Each of the campground descriptions includes ratings for beauty, site privacy, site spaciousness, quiet, security, and cleanliness; each attribute is ranked from one to five stars, with five being the best. Yes, these ratings are subjective, but we've tried to select campgrounds that offer something for everyone.

BEAUTY

Exceptional scenery can be found throughout Texas, but the five-star campgrounds will provide breathtaking views—you will know you're in a special place. The campground will be situated for full enjoyment of the view, which may be a towering mountain range or the perfect forest pond or stream.

SITE PRIVACY

Ideally, trees, shrubs, and other natural features will be left in place or incorporated into the site development to offer privacy and barriers between adjacent sites. The best campgrounds have well-spaced sites with little visual contact between neighbors and a sense of solitude due to the campground's distance from the nearest roads and towns.

QUIET

Our top rating for quiet means little or no overhead or road noise, minimal social noise, an aura of solitude, and quiet hours enforced by staff (if there is any staff). It was a plus if we could hear the water from a nearby river or stream, birds singing, or the wind through the trees. Quiet is a difficult attribute to quantify because we all know it can change quickly, depending on your neighbor.

SITE SPACIOUSNESS

Spacious to us means plenty of room for two tents to be set back from the parking area and away from the fire ring. There should also be space for separate areas to cook, eat, and just relax without being on top of your neighbors.

SECURITY

Many of the parks have an on-site host or park rangers regularly checking the campgrounds, and these have received higher ratings. The entrance stations were also staffed during daylight hours for increased security.

CLEANLINESS

Everyone wants to see clean restrooms, fire pits, and picnic tables and a campground free of ground litter. If the tent site was well maintained and the restrooms and showers were recently constructed, the campground received higher marks.

THE CAMPGROUND PROFILE

Each profile contains a concise but informative narrative that describes the campground and individual sites. Readers get a sense not only of the property itself but also the recreational opportunities available nearby. This descriptive text is enhanced with three helpful sidebars: Ratings, Key Information, and Getting There (accurate driving directions that lead you to the campground from the nearest major roadway).

THE CAMPGROUND LOCATOR MAP AND MAP LEGEND

Use the Texas Campground Locator Map, on page iv, to assess the exact location of each campground. The campground's number appears not only on the overview map but also in the table of contents and on the profile's first page.

A map legend that details the symbols found on the campground-layout maps appears on page vii.

CAMPGROUND-LAYOUT MAPS

Each profile contains a detailed map of campground sites, internal roads, facilities, and other key items.

GPS CAMPGROUND-ENTRANCE COORDINATES

Readers can easily access all campgrounds in this book by using the directions given and the overview map, which shows at least one major road leading into the area. But for those who enjoy using GPS technology to navigate, the book includes coordinates for each campground's entrance in latitude and longitude, expressed in degrees and decimal minutes.

To convert GPS coordinates from degrees, minutes, and seconds to the above degree decimal-minute format, the seconds are divided by 60. For more on GPS technology, visit usgs.gov.

A note of caution: Actual GPS devices will easily guide you to any of these campgrounds, but users of smartphone mapping apps may find that cell phone service is often unavailable in the remote areas where many of these hideaways are located.

ABOUT THIS BOOK

Whether you are a new arrival or a native Texan, it doesn't take long to recognize the size and diversity of the Lone Star State. From the High Plains of the Panhandle to the tropics of South Texas, the state stretches an amazing 906 miles from north to south. From the desert climate of El Paso to the towering piney woods of East Texas, a mere 841 miles will connect you. While this guidebook covers a lot of those miles, it is impossible to know every perfect tent campground, and I'm quite sure some were missed. In fact, there are probably many sites known only to the few who have had the good fortune to find them but wisely don't invite the entire state to join them in their special place of solitude. I understand and respect that. We all need that one secret place to escape to.

The good news is that Texas is so big that we can all find our own haven in the hills or valleys. Whether you love the deepest woods, the driest desert, the tallest mountain, or the unlimited seashore, this book will help you find a place to claim as your own.

WEATHER

In many parts of Texas, rain may come at any time, but keep in mind that weather patterns are most likely to change in the late afternoon. High winds may kick up with little warning, so stay alert if you're enjoying a day on the lakes or rivers. Spring or summer afternoons often bring intense rainstorms with lightning followed by spectacular sunsets. Overnight storms can also be a real surprise, so be sure to stake down your tent and put on your rainfly. Know what to do and how to seek safe shelter when these storms hit. In an emergency, use your car for immediate shelter, but be aware of low-water crossings and the danger of flash floods. Tornadoes also require special precautions, so know where to find the closest sturdy structure.

Of course, the weather is part of what makes Texas such a great place to camp, but it also provides its main danger—heat. As in many southwestern locations, a large number of Texas's best hiking trails not only provide a significant physical challenge but also the dangers of heat exhaustion and heat stroke. Don't be fooled by cool mornings or a few clouds. Always carry a hat, sunscreen, trail snacks, and more water than you might think you'll need. A good rule is 2–4 quarts per person per day, but even this is a bare minimum where temperatures may approach 100°F by noon. The best advice is to hike very early in the morning or late in the afternoon to avoid the brutal midday sun. Then spend the rest of the day under the trees or in a local spring-fed pond or river. Camping and hiking in Texas, even in summer, can be a highly rewarding experience if you respect the elements. Remember, even the rattlesnakes seek cover in the hot summer sun. You should do the same.

While Texas has a reputation for mild falls and winters, conditions from November to March can vary greatly, from snow in the High Plains, to ice storms in East Texas, and balmy temperatures along the Gulf Coast. Be sure to check up-to-date weather forecasts before any Texas adventures.

FIRST AID KIT

A useful first aid kit may contain more items than you might think necessary. These are just the basics. Prepackaged kits in waterproof bags (Atwater Carey and Adventure Medical Kits make them) are available. As a preventive measure, take along sunscreen and insect repellent. Even though quite a few items are listed here, they pack down into a small space:

- Ace bandages or Spenco joint wraps
- Adhesive bandages, such as Band-Aids
- Antibiotic ointment (Neosporin or the generic equivalent)
- Antiseptic or disinfectant, such as Betadine
- Aspirin, acetaminophen (Tylenol), or ibuprofen (Advil)
- Benadryl or the generic equivalent, diphenhydramine (in case of allergic reactions)
- Butterfly-closure bandages
- Comb and tweezers (for removing ticks from your skin)
- Epinephrine in a prefilled syringe (for severe allergic reactions to outdoor mishaps such as bee stings)
- Gauze (one roll and six 4-by-4-inch compress pads)
- LED flashlight or headlamp
- Matches or lighter
- Moist towelettes
- Moleskin/Spenco 2nd Skin
- Pocketknife or multipurpose tool
- Tick remover
- Tweezers
- Waterproof first aid tape
- Whistle (for signaling rescuers if you get lost or hurt)

ANIMAL AND PLANT HAZARDS

BEARS

The black bear is the only ursine species in Texas. It is on the state endangered species list, so it's rare that you'll see one, but to be safe keep your campsite clean and clear of food temptations. If you do encounter a bear, remain calm and back away slowly—*never* run. Make yourself look larger than you are by raising your arms or backpack above your head. If attacked, fight back with anything available.

MOUNTAIN LIONS

Stealthy and shy, the mountain lion is another animal you're unlikely to see despite its presence throughout West Texas. Should you encounter a mountain lion that doesn't immediately retreat, stand your ground. As with bears, make yourself look large, stick with your group, and make noise. Don't run—that makes the mountain lion's natural hunting instincts kick in. If the cat attacks, *fight.*

MOSQUITOES

Culex mosquitoes, the primary type that can transmit West Nile virus to humans, usually thrive in heavily populated urban areas. They lay their eggs in stagnant water and can breed in water that has been standing for more than five days. Although it happens only rarely, you can contract West Nile virus if you get bitten by an infected mosquito. Most people infected with West Nile have no symptoms of illness, but some may become ill, usually 3–15 days after being bitten. Protect yourself with an insect repellent that contains DEET as its active ingredient, and a good campfire helps protect you as you roast the marshmallows.

POISON IVY

Many Texas parks have healthy crops of poison ivy (*right*), which may grow along trails and in less-maintained sections of the camping areas. Learn to recognize the three-leaf pattern and steer clear! If you do get into a patch, washing the affected skin with alcohol, soap, and water can prevent the rash from developing. If you know you get the rash easily, always wear long pants when hiking through underbrush and carry an alcohol-based hand sanitizer and a washcloth. Be sure to eventually wash off shoes and anything else that may have the oil on it. If you are exposed to poison ivy, raised lines or blisters will usually appear within 12 hours (but sometimes much later), accompanied by

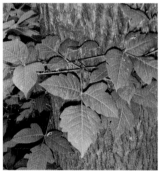

photo: *Tom Watson*

a terrible itch. Refrain from scratching because it can cause infection, but it won't spread the rash, as is commonly believed. Wash and dry the area thoroughly. Various over-the-counter products will alleviate the symptoms until it heals on its own. In the worse cases, a doctor can prescribe treatment.

SNAKES

Be extra alert in any outdoor setting in Texas for not only rattlesnakes but also copperheads and a few other snakes such as coral snakes and water moccasins. Your best defense is to watch where you step or reach, and when you do see a snake, or any wild animal, leave it alone. They're often just as unhappy to see you, so go around and let them be.

As with any outdoor activity in Texas, watch for fire ants, spiders, and occasional scorpions.

CAMPING TIPS

Car camping is a great way to see Texas. It offers the flexibility to stay places where others may not tread without forcing you to strap on a backpack. As you explore, please use camping techniques that will minimize your impact on the sites you use. Like the efforts of a careful backcountry camper, using these techniques will leave the site in good condition for the next person to enjoy.

Here are a few things to consider as you prepare for your trip:

- **PLAN AHEAD.** Know your equipment, your ability, and the area where you are camping—and prepare accordingly. Be self-sufficient at all times; carry the necessary supplies for changes in weather or other conditions. A well-executed trip is satisfying.

- **USE CARE WHEN TRAVELING.** Stay on designated roadways. Be respectful of private property and travel restrictions. Familiarize yourself with the area you'll be traveling in by picking up a map that shows land ownership. Such maps are typically available from U.S. Forest Service offices for a small fee.

- **RESERVE YOUR SITE IN ADVANCE,** especially if it's a weekend or a holiday, or if the campground is wildly popular. Many prime campgrounds require at least a six-month lead time on reservations. Check before you go.

  When selecting a site, consider your space requirements and match the site to your needs. Try to keep your group size small. If you're traveling in a large group, consider splitting up so that no more than eight people are at a single campsite. Wear and tear on a site with a large group of people can be significant even if you stay only a short time.

- **CHECK IN, PAY YOUR FEE, AND MARK YOUR SITE AS DIRECTED.** Don't just grab a seemingly empty site that looks more appealing than yours—it could be reserved. If you're unhappy with the site you've selected, check with the campground host for other options.

- **PICK YOUR CAMPING BUDDIES WISELY.** A family trip is pretty straightforward, but you may want to reconsider including grumpy Uncle Fred, who doesn't like bugs, sunshine, or marshmallows. After you know who's going, make sure that everyone is on the same page regarding expectations of difficulty (amenities or the lack thereof, physical exertion, and so on), sleeping arrangements, and food requirements.

- **DRESS FOR THE SEASON.** Educate yourself on the temperature highs and lows of the specific part of the state you plan to visit. It may be warm at night in the summer in your backyard, but up in the mountains it will be quite chilly.

- **PITCH YOUR TENT ON A LEVEL SURFACE,** preferably one covered with leaves, pine straw, or grass. Use a tarp or specially designed footprint to thwart ground moisture and to protect the tent floor. Do a little site maintenance, such as picking up the small rocks and sticks that can damage your tent floor and make sleeping uncomfortable. If you have a separate tent rain-fly but don't think you'll need it, keep it rolled up at the base of the tent in case it starts raining at midnight.

- **CONSIDER TAKING A SLEEPING PAD** if the ground makes you uncomfortable. Choose a pad that is full length and thicker than you think you might need. This will not only keep your hips from aching on hard ground, but it will also help keep you warm. A wide range of thin, light, or inflatable pads is available at camping stores, and these are a much better choice than home air mattresses, which conduct heat away from the body and tend to deflate during the night.

- **DON'T HANG OR TIE CLOTHESLINES, HAMMOCKS, AND EQUIPMENT TO OR FROM TREES.** You may see this being commonly practiced in many developed campgrounds, but be responsible and do your part to reduce damage to trees and shrubs.

- **IF YOU TEND TO USE THE BATHROOM MULTIPLE TIMES AT NIGHT, PLAN AHEAD.** Leaving a warm sleeping bag and stumbling around in the dark to find the restroom—be it a pit toilet, a fully plumbed comfort station, or just the woods—is not fun. Keep a flashlight and any other accoutrements you may need by the tent door, and know exactly where to head in the dark.

- **WHEN YOU CAMP AT A DISPERSED SITE, KNOW HOW TO GO.** The lack of toilet facilities and water is the biggest challenge. Bringing large filled water jugs and a portable toilet are the easiest and most environmentally friendly solutions.

  Many portable toilets are available from outdoor-supply catalogs; in a pinch, a 5-gallon bucket fixed with a toilet seat and lined with a heavy-duty plastic trash bag will work just as well. (Be sure to pack out the trash bag.)

  A second, less desirable method is to dig 8-inch-deep catholes. These should be located at least 200 yards from campsites, trails, and water and in inconspicuous locations with as much undergrowth as possible. (Be creative and find spots with a great view—just make sure you aren't providing a great view for others!) Cover the hole with a thin layer of soil after each use, and do not burn or bury your toilet paper—pack it out in resealable plastic bags. If you'll be in the campsite for several days, dig a new hole each day, being careful to replace the topsoil over the hole from the day before.

  In addition to the plastic bags, your outdoor-toilet cache should include a garden trowel, toilet paper, and premoistened towelettes. Select a trowel with a well-designed handle that can also double as a toilet paper dispenser.

- **IF YOU AREN'T HIKING TO A PRIMITIVE CAMPSITE, DON'T SKIMP ON FOOD.** Plan tasty meals, and bring everything you'll need to prepare, cook, eat, and clean up. That said, don't duplicate equipment such as cooking pots among the members of your group. Carry what you need, but don't turn the trip into a cross-country moving experience.

- **KEEP A CLEAN KITCHEN AREA,** and avoid leaving food scraps on the ground both during and after your visit. Maintain a group trash bag, and be sure to secure it in your vehicle or a bear-proof food locker at night. Many sites have a pack-in/pack-out rule, and that means everything: no cheating by tossing orange peels, eggshells, or apple cores in the shrubs.

- **DO YOUR PART TO HELP PREVENT BEARS FROM BECOMING CONDITIONED TO SEEKING HUMAN FOOD.** The constant search for food influences every aspect of a bear's life, so while camping in bear country, store food in your vehicle or in site-provided bear-proof boxes. Keep food (including canned goods, soft drinks, and beer) and garbage secured, and resist the temptation to take food into your tent. You'll also need to stow scented or flavored toiletries such as toothpaste and lip balm, as well as cooking grease and pet food. Common sense and adherence to the simple rules posted at the campgrounds will help keep you and the bears safe and healthy. (See page 4 for what to do if you encounter a bear.)

- **USE ESTABLISHED FIRE RINGS, AND ALWAYS INQUIRE ABOUT CURRENT FIRE RESTRICTIONS.** Don't burn garbage in your campfire—trash often doesn't burn completely, and fire rings fill with burned litter over time. Be sure your fire is totally extinguished when you leave the area. If you cook with a Dutch oven, be sure to use a fire pan, and elevate it to avoid scorching or burning the ground.

  Note that many campground operators frown upon bringing your own firewood from home, so check ahead to see if it's allowed. Bringing in wood from outside of the area could introduce pests that are harmful to the forest, so if it's prohibited by the campground you plan to visit, use deadfall found near your campsite—again, only if permitted—or purchase wood at the camp store.

- **DON'T BATHE OR WASH DISHES AND LAUNDRY IN STREAMS AND LAKES.** Food scraps are unsightly and can be potentially harmful to fish, and even biodegradable soap can be harmful to fragile aquatic environments.

- **BE COURTEOUS TO OTHER CAMPERS.** Observe quiet hours, keep noise to a minimum, and keep pets leashed and under control.

- **MOST IMPORTANT, PLEASE LEAVE YOUR CAMP CLEANER THAN YOU FOUND IT.** Pick up all trash and microlitter in your site, including in your fire ring. Disperse leftover brush used for firewood.

Now that your head is full of facts, pick up the crew, purchase a Texas State Parks Pass ($70) or a National Parks & Federal Recreation Lands Annual Pass ($80) for one year of unlimited free entrance fees, and enjoy the best tent camping in the Lone Star State. These passes are available at most entrance stations or visitor centers and provide the best way to enjoy and share the 50 special places described for you and your family.

BIG BEND COUNTRY AND THE GUADALUPE MOUNTAINS

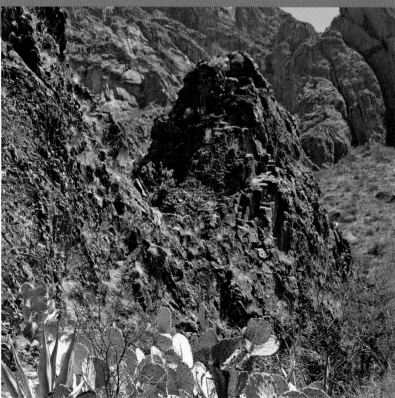

No level tent sites here (Big Bend National Park: Chisos Basin Campground; see page 16)

⚠ Abilene State Park

Beauty: ★★★ / Privacy: ★★★ / Spaciousness: ★★★ / Quiet: ★★★ / Security: ★★★★ / Cleanliness: ★★★

Buffalo Gap Historic Village takes you back in time to an era when tent camping was not recreational.

Located at the crossroads of Texas history, Abilene State Park is surrounded by low lime-stone hills in a rugged area used first by the Tonkawa and Comanche to hunt buffalo and later by Texas cowboys leading cattle drives on the Goodnight–Loving Trail. On your way to the park, a stop at the restored Buffalo Gap Historic Village (325-572-3365) takes you back in time to an era when tent camping was not recreational but required for traveling across the vastness of West Texas; the legendary Butterfield stage route went through this area in the mid-19th century. This line of early communication ran through the hunting grounds of several American Indian tribes who recognized that these latest arrivals were a serious threat to their way of life. The name Buffalo Gap refers to a break in the hills used by migrating buffalo. The local tribesmen's dependence on the buffalo ultimately hastened their downfall as the Texas Longhorn replaced the vast herds of buffalo.

As you leave headquarters on the Panhandle Plains Wildlife Trail, the first right turn leads to the swimming pool area and beautiful rock structures built in 1933 by Civilian Conservation Corps (CCC) Company 1823, consisting of World War I veterans who found themselves unemployed during the Great Depression. In 1935 this company also included black veterans, a CCC first in Texas. Be sure to examine the water tower, pool buildings, and picnic areas to appreciate the workmanship and heavy labor of these former soldiers.

Returning toward the main road, stay right at the fork toward Cedar Grove tent camp-ground on your left. This small campground is hidden in a thick grove of evergreen cedars that provides not only welcome shade, but more important, protection from the West Texas wind. While all the sites are good, look for sites 39, 40, and 42 at the back of the circle drive. These sites have a little more space and back up to some heavy brush and a dry creekbed. The sites are also within a short walk to the large family-friendly swimming pool.

Dry dock in winter—wet fun in summer

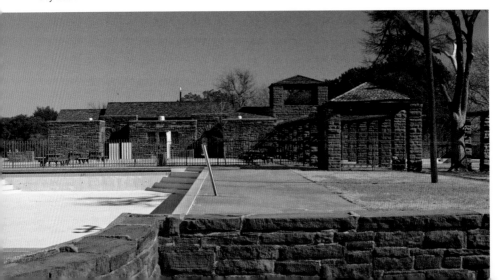

KEY INFORMATION

ADDRESS: 150 Park Road 32, Tuscola, TX 79562

CONTACT: 325-572-3204, tpwd.texas.gov/state-parks/abilene

OPERATED BY: Texas Parks & Wildlife Department

OPEN: Year-round

SITES: 12 in Cedar Grove, 21 in Pecan Grove

EACH SITE: Picnic table, fire ring, lantern hook, central water

ASSIGNMENT: First come, first served until site-specific reservation system begins in 2018

REGISTRATION: At headquarters or reserve at texas.reserveworld.com or 512-389-8900

FACILITIES: Swimming pool, modern restrooms

PARKING: At each site

FEE: $12/night at Cedar Grove (water only); $15/night at Pecan Grove; $5/person entrance fee, age 12 and under free

ELEVATION: 1,993'

RESTRICTIONS:

PETS: On leash only

FIRES: Fire rings only; check on burn bans

ALCOHOL: Prohibited in all public/outdoor areas

VEHICLES: 2/site

OTHER: Maximum 8 people/site; guests must leave by 10 p.m.; quiet time 10 p.m.– 6 a.m.; bring your own firewood or charcoal; limited supplies at Buffalo Gap; pick up main supplies in Abilene; gathering firewood prohibited

Returning to the main road, turn right and watch for the numerous armadillos poking around for a snack. Travel 0.8 mile into the heart of the park over low-water crossings to Pecan Grove sites 62–84. This area has electricity and some RVs, but the massive pecan trees shade most of the sites, which also have large, level tent pads. Look for sites 74, 75, and 79 for the most privacy and easy access to the Elm Creek Nature Trail and the Eagle Trail.

As you leave the park, turn left on FM 89 for access to Lake Abilene, along with a close-up view of massive wind farms generating clean electricity from that always-reliable West Texas wind still carrying the history of westward expansion.

VOICES FROM THE CAMPFIRE AND RECOMMENDED READING

The foundations of the state park system enjoyed by Texans today were laid in the bittersweet years of the 1930s. The Great Depression's hardships inspired many public works programs for the unemployed after 1929, and park development became a popular means of relief.

With Franklin D. Roosevelt's inauguration as president in March 1933, his New Deal elevated conservation and public recreation to a national crusade. . . . Recruits enrolled for six-month periods and received $30 per month. Selected men were paid $36 and $45 per month as clerks, cooks, and leaders. At least $25 of the monthly wage was sent directly to the CCC worker's family back home.

James Wright Steely, *The Civilian Conservation Corps in Texas State Parks* (Austin, Texas Parks & Wildlife Department, 2010).

BACKCOUNTRY ADVENTURES

Canoe or kayak across Lake Abilene and hike into the hills to the north for amazing views. Boat rentals are available in the park.

BEST LOCAL FOOD AND DRINK

Perini Ranch Steakhouse (325-572-3339; store.periniranch.com) in Buffalo Gap is one of the best restaurants in the state. Beehive Restaurant (325-675-0600; beehivesaloon.com) in Abilene has lots of cold beer, cocktails, and traditional Texas fare.

Abilene State Park

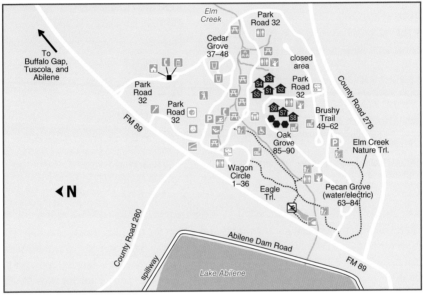

GETTING THERE

From Abilene, drive about 16 miles southwest on FM 89/Buffalo Gap Road. Turn left onto Park Road 32 to reach the entrance.

GPS COORDINATES:
  N32° 14.448' W99° 52.734'

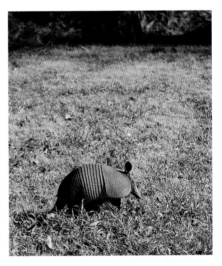

A Texas icon—the armadillo

Balmorhea State Park

Beauty: ★★ / Privacy: ★★ / Spaciousness: ★★★ / Quiet: ★★ / Security: ★★★★ / Cleanliness: ★★★

This incredible spring rewards travelers with a 22-foot-deep swimmer's paradise.

Note: The park's camping and lodging are undergoing major repairs until early 2019. Contact the park for reopening dates for these areas.

After leaving the scenic Davis Mountains, TX 17 returns to the wide-open, hot, and very dry expanses of West Texas, only to be interrupted by a hidden oasis that surprises even a well-traveled tent camper. As you approach the entrance station, there is little to indicate a special location other than a full parking lot, swimsuits, and swimmers of every size and shape, and panel trucks from SCUBA shops all over Texas. This small state park is home to San Solomon Springs and has provided lifesaving water to American Indians, Spanish explorers, frontier soldiers, and myriad Texas travelers. Beginning in the 1930s, the Civilian Conservation Corps built a 2-acre swimming pool with an underground source of crystal-clear 75°F water flowing at nearly 20 million gallons per day. This incredible spring rewards travelers with a 22-foot-deep swimmer's paradise. The pool also serves as an ideal training ground for novice SCUBA divers looking for a safe practice spot before heading to the open ocean. The pool has the added benefit of being chlorine free, due to the constant inflow and outflow of this artesian spring.

A rare West Texas oasis

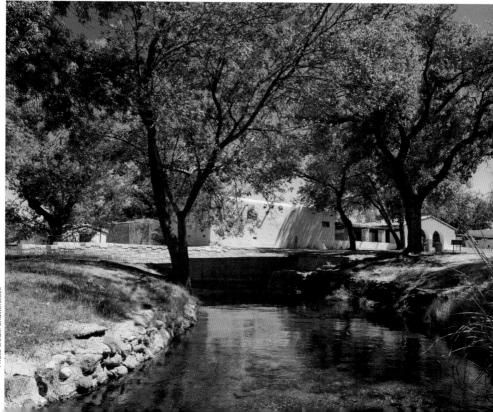

Photo credit: *Shutterstock*

KEY INFORMATION

ADDRESS: 9207 TX 17, Toyahvale, TX 79786

CONTACT: 432-375-2370,
tpwd.texas.gov/state-parks/balmorhea

OPERATED BY: Texas Parks & Wildlife
Department

OPEN: Year-round (see note on page 13
regarding renovations)

SITES: 32

EACH SITE: Water

ASSIGNMENT: First come, first served
until site-specific reservation system
begins in 2018

REGISTRATION: At headquarters/entrance
station or reserve at texas.reserveworld
.com or 512-389-8900

FACILITIES: Picnic tables, covered shelters,
fire rings, upright charcoal grills

PARKING: At each site

FEE: $11 for tent sites; $7/person entrance fee

ELEVATION: 3,248'

RESTRICTIONS:

PETS: On leash only

FIRES: Check for burn bans during dry
weather

ALCOHOL: Prohibited in all public/outdoor
areas

VEHICLES: 2/site

OTHER: Maximum 8 people/site; guests must
leave by 10 p.m.; quiet time 10 p.m.–
6 a.m.; bring your own firewood or charcoal; limited supplies at park store; pick up
necessities in Toyahvale, Fort Davis, or
Pecos; gathering firewood prohibited

After leaving the pool, the water flows by small canal into a newly restored ciénaga, or desert wetland, that is home to the endangered Pecos gambusia and Comanche Springs pupfish. Destroyed by the construction of the pool in the 1930s, this area is now being restored by Texas Parks & Wildlife and other partners to its original location and function as a living ecosystem downstream from the pool area. Given its location in a desert, the vegetation is also truly unique, including cattails, rushes, and reeds.

The campground begins just to the left of the pool parking lot and contains RV sites until sites 14–19 in the back, right corner. These spacious sites hold a number of tents. It's not exactly a wilderness experience, but the miracle of water in the desert will help your body recover from those mountain hikes in Big Bend, the Davis Mountains, or Guadalupe Peak, which surround this little-known but refreshing watering hole. The wide-open views and lack of wind breaks around this campground will require some extra staking, but a visit to this two-acre swimming pool in summer is well worth it. Be sure to bring your lawn chairs, swimming gear, and sun protection so you won't suffer overnight in your tent. Also, be aware that while the summer days can easily exceed 100°F, nights cool off quickly.

VOICES FROM THE CAMPFIRE AND RECOMMENDED READING

In the hunting and gathering way of life, the whole territory of a given group is fairly equally experienced by everyone. Those wild and sacred spots have many uses. There are places where women go for seclusion, places where the bodies of the dead are taken, and spots where young men and women are called for special instruction. Such places are numinous, loaded with meaning and power. The memories of such spots are very long.
Gary Snyder, *The Practice of the Wild* (Berkeley, CA, Counterpoint Press, 2010).

BACKCOUNTRY ADVENTURES

This park is a mecca for all levels of SCUBA divers and snorkelers. Those interested in SCUBA diving should bring their own equipment and proof of certification, and have a buddy to accompany them during their dives.

BEST LOCAL FOOD AND DRINK

Bear Den (Mexican food) (432-375-2273) and Juan Carrasco Mercantile (general menu, TV) (432-375-0240) in Balmorhea. Circle Bar & Saddleback Steakhouse (432-755-4380) is also a local favorite, located near I-10 and TX 17.

Balmorhea State Park

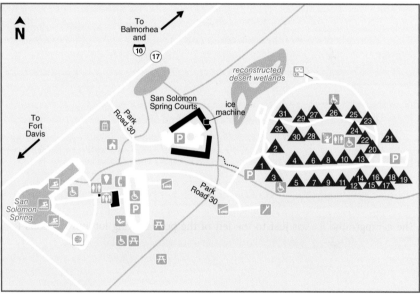

GETTING THERE

From Fort Davis, travel north on TX 17 for about 32 miles. The park entrance will be on the right.

From I-10, exit onto TX 17 and travel south about 7 miles. The park entrance will be on the left.

GPS COORDINATES: N30° 56.682' W103° 46.200'

Big Bend National Park:

CHISOS BASIN CAMPGROUND

Beauty: ★★★★★ / Privacy: ★★ / Spaciousness: ★★ / Quiet: ★★★ / Security: ★★★★ / Cleanliness: ★★★★

Limited tent sites and a little noise pollution are small prices to pay for the breathtaking landscape on all sides.

With a captivating panoramic view of the Chisos Mountains, Chisos Basin Campground is one of the most popular camping areas in Big Bend National Park. Turning right off the main park road, a winding road leads into the campground. Follow the road by keeping to the left until the "no generator zone" begins around site 48. Although there are a handful of acceptable tent sites in 1–47, the best sites are 48–60. Site 59 is secluded, with relaxing shade and an excellent view of the surrounding peaks, while site 60 is quite spacious, perfect for a family or small group. Site 55 is hidden from the road and has its own trail to the restroom. If you're here to explore the park, any site will do if you arrive late and don't get your first choice. After choosing your location, feed the pay station, and begin your exploration of one of the most remote and scenic national parks in the country.

There are many hiking trails in Big Bend, and some of the best are near the Chisos Basin area. Most notably, the Window Trail has one of its trailheads located in the campground itself. With a round-trip of 5.6 miles and a moderate uphill return, the trail is well worth the

Tent camping on the edge of nothing . . . and everything

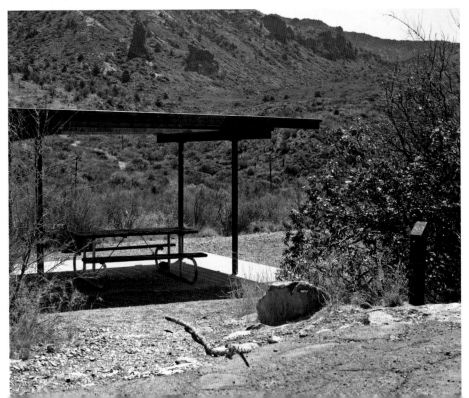

KEY INFORMATION

ADDRESS: Window View Dr., Big Bend National Park, TX 79834

OPERATED BY: National Park Service

CONTACT: 432-477-2251, nps.gov/bibe; reservations: 877-444-6777, recreation.gov

OPEN: Year-round

SITES: 60 individual, 7 group

EACH SITE: Picnic tables, bear box

ASSIGNMENT: First come, first served (26 sites can be reserved Nov 15–May 31)

REGISTRATION: Self-pay station

FACILITIES: Flush toilets, centrally located drinking water, dishwashing sink, showers at Rio Grande Village Campground only

PARKING: At campsites and next to restrooms

FEE: $7–$14/night, group site $27; entrance fee $25/vehicle/7 day, $50 Big Bend Annual Pass

ELEVATION: 5,401'

RESTRICTIONS:

PETS: On leash only

FIRES: No ground fires or wood fires allowed. Designated smoking bans may also be in effect.

ALCOHOL: Prohibited in most areas; see rules at nps.gov/bibe/planyourvisit/alcoholpolicy.htm

VEHICLES: Cars, vans, trailers, RVs; tent camping only in "no generator zone"

OTHER: Maximum 8 people/site; quiet time: 10 p.m.–6 a.m.; 14-day camping limit; no smoking on trails

effort to see the postcard-worthy Window View. Other trails in the area include the Lost Mine and Basin Loop. Near the other trailhead to the Window Trail and Basin Loop are the visitor center, store, restaurant, and lodge. The visitor center is informative and includes current information on weather, trail conditions, and animal sightings/warnings. Also check for trail, campsite, and climbing area closures or restrictions done seasonally to protect the popular nesting areas of the peregrine falcon. See the park's Daily Report for up-to-date conditions.

Wildlife around the campground is quite diverse. Mammals include the piglike javelinas, jackrabbits, skunks, black bears, and even mountain lions. Ask a ranger or read the numerous signs to find out what to do if you encounter a bear or mountain lion. Also, be sure to use the bear box to store all food and scented items, and keep a clean campsite.

Chisos Basin Campground is the most highly visited campground in Big Bend, thanks to the rugged mountains and relatively cool temperatures. Therefore, the campsites fill up quickly and campers seeking to get away from the hustle and bustle of the city may feel a little too close to their neighbor. However, the limited number of tent sites and a little noise pollution are a small price to pay for the breathtaking landscape on all sides and the kaleidoscope of stars at night. So special are night skies at Big Bend that it's one of the few official Dark Sky Parks in the world.

VOICES FROM THE CAMPFIRE AND RECOMMENDED READING

The scene is set. — According to Indian legend, when the Great Creator made the earth and had finished placing the stars in the sky, the birds in the air, and the fish in the sea, there was a large pile of rejected stony materials left over. Finished with His job, He threw this into one heap and made the Big Bend.

Ross A. Maxwell, *The Big Bend of the Rio Grande: A Guide to the Rocks, Landscape, Geologic History, and Settlers of the Area of Big Bend National Park* (Austin, University of Texas, 1968).

BACKCOUNTRY ADVENTURES

A multitude of unique and diverse wonders can be experienced while exploring Big Bend National Park. Treat yourself to the rare beauty of the cactus bloom during a spring desert hike, the fall colors along Bonita Springs canyon, and the stunning view from the edge of the south rim. For those wanting more of a challenge, climb to the top of Emory Peak, the highest point in the park. Visit several times and find your own favorite spot.

BEST LOCAL FOOD AND DRINK

The restaurant inside the Chisos Mountains Lodge (877-386-4383; chisosmountainslodge .com) offers a full menu, bar, and patio with tables and chairs to watch the stunning sunsets. You can also preorder a sack lunch and enjoy a buffet breakfast, which is great for filling up before a long hike. The small camp store next to the visitor center carries staples, including snacks, drinks, and ice cream. The surrounding historical communities of Marathon, Study Butte, and Terlingua offer wonderful dining but are several miles away from the park, so plan accordingly. Filling up your stomach, gas tank, and supplies takes planning in this remote area.

Big Bend National Park: Chisos Basin Campground

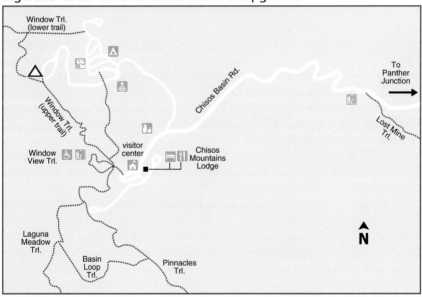

GETTING THERE

From Marathon, go south on US 385. Proceed past the Persimmon Gap Visitor Center and turn right at Panther Junction. Keep traveling 3 miles until you get to the Chisos Mountains Basin Junction, and turn left. Follow the road 7 miles until you come to the Chisos Basin Campground. Turn right and follow the road to the campground. Stay to the left until you see the "no generator zone" and tent sites 49–60.

GPS COORDINATES: N29° 16.518' W103° 18.060'

4

Big Bend National Park: RIO GRANDE
VILLAGE AND COTTONWOOD CAMPGROUNDS

Beauty: ★★★★ / Privacy: ★★★ / Spaciousness: ★★★ / Quiet: ★★ / Security: ★★ / Cleanliness: ★★★★

In winter, don't miss the incredible bird-watching opportunities here.

Leaving the cool, dry air of the Chisos Basin area, the 30-mile drive to the Rio Grande Village Campground takes the tent camper through 3,600 feet of elevation loss and expanses of the Chihuahuan Desert that appear endless, with the drive ending with an arrival in a shaded oasis that seems almost tropical. While the campground is on a level area adjacent to the Rio Grande, the opposite side of the river contains massive limestone rock formations in the area known as Boquillas Canyon. After entering the campground, look for the non-generator zone in the back. These sites are shielded by heavy vegetation; sites 22–30 offer the most privacy. Also, search out sites 16–19 for nice locations for covered tables and tents.

When considering camping at Rio Grande Village, be aware that temperatures from May to September are probably not pleasant for tent camping, but winter months allow not only for good overnight stays but also for incredible bird-watching opportunities in an area with more than 450 confirmed species. The joy of desert hiking is also greater in the wintertime. If a cold blast does come through, however, be sure to visit the hot springs located 1.9 miles off the park road as you approach the main campground and park store. Another worthwhile side trip is the 4-mile drive to Boquillas Canyon Overlook and the Rio Grande as it turns almost north to complete the big bend that gives this national park its name. A final note on visiting this area of the park: Remember that the traditional informal crossing of the river to visit and trade with Mexico was previously strictly prohibited, then reopened, and the future status is unknown. Be sure to check with park officials before attempting to cross under any circumstances.

The joy and beauty of high desert travel

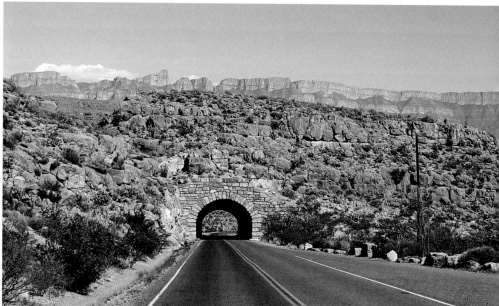

KEY INFORMATION

ADDRESS: Rio Grande Village RV Campground: Big Bend National Park, TX 79834 (20 miles east from Panther Junction entrance)
Cottonwood Campground: Big Bend National Park, TX 79834 (36 miles southwest of Panther Junction Visitor Center)

OPERATED BY: National Park Service

CONTACT: 915-477-2251, nps.gov/bibe; reservations: 915-477-2291 for non-RV information, recreation.gov

OPEN: Year-round

SITES: 93: 1 group walk-in in Cottonwood, 4 group sites in Rio Grande Village

EACH SITE: Picnic table, grill, bear box

ASSIGNMENT: Reservations get you in the campground; site choice is first come, first served

REGISTRATION: Self-pay station

FACILITIES: Flush toilets, drinking water, showers, washer/dryer near park store (open year-round)

PARKING: At each site

FEE: $7–$14/night, group site $27; entrance fee $25/vehicle/7 day; $50 annual pass (Big Bend)

ELEVATION: 1,830'

RESTRICTIONS:

PETS: On leash only

FIRES: Charcoal and stoves only; no ground or wood fires

ALCOHOL: Prohibited in most areas; see rules at nps.gov/bibe/planyourvisit/alcoholpolicy.htm

VEHICLES: 2/site

OTHER: Maximum 8 people/site; quiet time: 8 p.m.–8 a.m.; bring your own charcoal; limited supplies available at park stores; pick up main supplies in Marathon or Fort Stockton; gathering firewood prohibited; visitor center closed May–October

---

Return on the main park road toward the Chisos Mountains Junction and continue straight to enjoy more wide-open spaces in Big Bend National Park. This well-paved but lightly traveled road takes you to some of the most scenic parts of the park. However, if you are looking for primitive campsites, dirt roads to your right will take you to Government Spring, Grapevine Spring, Paint Gap, and Croton Spring campgrounds. Be sure to inquire at the Panther Junction Visitor Center about road conditions or any other helpful information about these remote desert areas.

Back on the main road, turn left at the Castolon/Santa Elena Junction and view the Chisos Mountains towering on your left. Also, take notice of the Sam Nail Ranch and Homer Wilson Ranch and try to imagine the hardships these early settlers faced. Just walking the short trail to the Wilson Ranch is a history lesson in desert survival. Likewise stop at Sotol Vista Overlook and Mule Ears Viewpoint to experience a landscape some may view as a barren expanse, but is one that contains a wide variety of flora whose beauty is only enhanced by the toughness necessary to thrive in this arid region. If you visit in spring and early summer, the display of flowering prickly pear cactus, desert willow, ocotillo, and yucca will have your cameras out to record the surprises in this barren world.

As you pass the Castolon Visitor Center (which is closed in summer) and the park store (open year-round), proceed 0.8 mile to the Cottonwood Campground turnoff on your left. This open expanse of a campground does not provide much privacy, and the tents are mixed with the RVs and trailers. However, the central area does provide an area of trees and grass for tents. There is also a resident band of javelinas known to assist with cleaning up the camp, should you forget to do so. This campground sits right on the Rio Grande and is a winter home for bird-watchers from around the world.

As if to make up for the absence of private tent-camping sites, leave the campground and continue 8 miles along the main road toward Santa Elena Canyon, one of the more famous sites in the National Park System of the United States. Take the Santa Elena Canyon Trail across a sandy creekbed and get a great view of the river as it emerges from between sheer 1,500-foot cliffs. This trail is less than 1 mile in length, but hiking it is a great way to end a trip to Big Bend or just to whet your appetite for more desert camping under the stars and the shade of towering cacti.

VOICES FROM THE CAMPFIRE AND RECOMMENDED READING

I made our bed in a dusty clearing in the cactus, but my beloved refused to sleep with me, preferring, she said, to curl up in the back seat of her car. The omens multiplied and all were dark. I slept alone under the shooting stars of Texas, dreaming of rocks and shovels.
Edward Abbey, *The Journey Home: Some Words in Defense of the American West* (New York, Dutton, 1977).

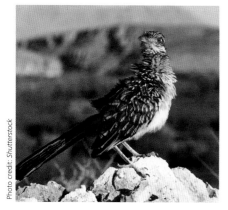

Photo credit: Shutterstock

Tough country, tough bird

"Chapter 3: Disorder and Early Sorrow" of *The Journey Home* contains the perfect description of ill-advised back-road travel in Big Bend starting near Castolon and Cottonwood Campground.

No more cars in national parks. Let the people walk. . . . We have agreed not to drive our automobiles into cathedrals, concert halls, art museums, legislative assemblies, private bedrooms and the other sanctums of our culture; we should treat our national parks with the same deference, for they, too, are holy places.
Edward Abbey, *Desert Solitaire: A Season in the Wilderness* (New York, McGraw-Hill, 1968).

BACKCOUNTRY ADVENTURES

The lower elevations of Big Bend National Park are world-famous bird-watching destinations. Raft trips down the Rio Grande can be a true adventure for even first-timers. Just be sure to drive carefully on the winding park roads, especially after dark.

BEST LOCAL FOOD AND DRINK

Within walking distance of the Rio Grande Village campground is a camp store with supplies, food, and drinks. Surrounding historical communities including Marathon, Study Butte, and Terlingua offer wonderful dining options but are several miles outside the park, so plan accordingly. This is one destination where you'll be glad you overpacked when it comes to food and water.

Big Bend National Park: Rio Grande Village Campground

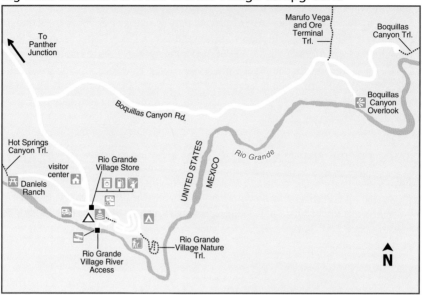

Big Bend National Park: Cottonwood Campground

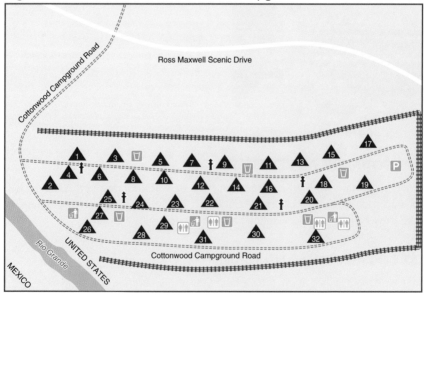

GETTING THERE

RIO GRANDE VILLAGE CAMPGROUND: From the intersection of US 385 and US 90 (near Marathon, TX), take US 385 S and drive 39.8 miles. Continue onto Main Park Road, past the Persimmon Gap Visitor Center, and continue 27.5 miles. Turn left onto Park Route 12 (when you see the Panther Junction Visitor Center in front of you), and drive 20.3 miles. Turn left and follow signs to the campground.

GPS COORDINATES: N29° 10.950' W102° 57.650'

COTTONWOOD CAMPGROUND (CASTALON): From the intersection of US 385 and US 90 (near Marathon, TX), take US 385 S and drive 39.8 miles. Continue onto Main Park Road, past the Persimmon Gap Visitor Center, and continue 27.5 miles. Turn right onto Gano Springs (when you see the Panther Junction Visitor Center in front of you), and drive 12.7 miles. Turn left onto Ross Maxwell Scenic Dr. (signs for Castalon) and drive 21.9 miles. Continue straight onto Santa Elena Canyon Road and drive 1.3 miles. Turn left and follow signs for Cottonwood Campground.

GPS COORDINATES: N29° 10.848' W102° 57.420'

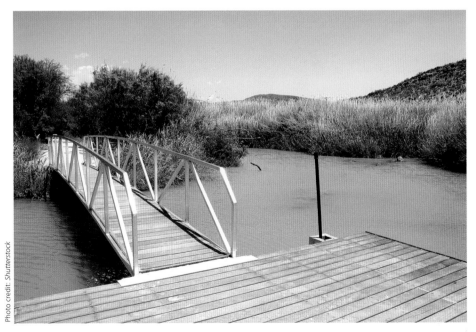

Photo credit: Shutterstock

At Big Bend National Park, you'll find great access to wildlife viewing.

5

Big Bend Ranch State Park

Beauty: ★★★★ / Privacy: ★★★ / Spaciousness: ★★★★ / Quiet: ★★★ / Security: ★★ / Cleanliness: ★★★

Be on the lookout for wild animals, such as deer and javelinas, which live in this wonderfully remote park.

Located in the shadow of its better-known neighbor, Big Bend Ranch State Park is an idyllic escape for those seeking a tent-camping site along the scenic Rio Grande with easy access to FM 170. Whether you're coming from Presidio to the northwest or Lajitas and Big Bend National Park to the southeast, the rugged beauty of this seldom-traveled road as it cuts through Colorado Canyon makes up for any lack of fancy campground amenities along the river. This road makes numerous low-water crossings. Be on the lookout for loose livestock, rockslides, and wild animals such as deer and javelinas, which live in this wonderfully remote park. It's also home to eagles, falcons, and migrating birds that come for the mild winters along the river. If you're looking for even more solitude and a true desert experience, bring your four-wheel drive or other high-clearance vehicle and travel to the interior of the 300,000 acres on Casa Piedra Road/FM 169. This 30-mile stretch of roadway will lead you to 12 primitive sites with hiking, mountain biking, and equestrian trails. There are showers near the historic lodge and Bunk House at Sauceda, but be sure to check in with the park to make sure they're accessible to primitive campers. The campsites have no water or electricity, so bring all needed supplies. You'll be rewarded with a wilderness experience and solitude usually reserved for backpackers.

The rewards of tent camping!

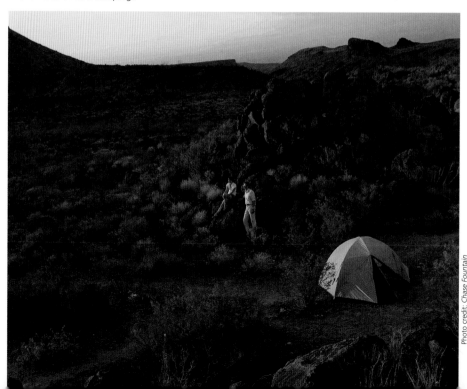

Photo credit: Chase Fountain

KEY INFORMATION

ADDRESS: 1900 Sauceda Ranch Road, Presidio, TX 79845

CONTACT: 432-358-4444, tpwd.texas.gov/state-parks/big-bend-ranch

OPERATED BY: Texas Parks & Wildlife Department

OPEN: Year-round

SITES: 47 in the southern portion of park, 66 interior sites. No designated group site, but some are close to each other and group friendly.

EACH SITE: Table, shelter, fire ring

ASSIGNMENT: First come, first served until site-specific reservation system begins in 2018

REGISTRATION: Barton Warnock Education Center or Fort Leaton State Historic Site; reserve at texas.reserveworld.com or 512-389-8900

FACILITIES: Chemical toilets along the river

PARKING: At each site

FEE: $5 (November–April), $3 (May–October)/ person, plus $8 camping fee

ELEVATION: 2,376'

RESTRICTIONS:

PETS: On leash only

FIRES: In fire rings only

ALCOHOL: Prohibited in all public/ outdoor areas

VEHICLES: 2/site

OTHER: Maximum 8 people/site; guests must leave by 10 p.m.; quiet time 10 p.m.– 6 a.m.; bring your own firewood or charcoal; limited supplies in Lajitas; pick up main supplies in Presidio; gathering firewood prohibited

Returning to FM 170, scan the rocky hillsides for herds of desert mountain goats traveling these steep heights with incredible ease. The main tent campgrounds are located at Colorado Canyon, Madera Canyon, and Grassy Banks. These sites also offer river access for the large number of rafters and canoe groups that wait patiently for the water level to rise. However, always call ahead if you're counting on a river trip—this desert river is unpredictable, but worth the wait.

As you travel along FM 170, the lush greenery along the banks contrasts starkly with the rugged cliffs towering above. All three campgrounds are adjacent to the river and benefit from the only shade within miles. The sandy soil also makes for a soft tent floor, and there is a compost toilet at each location. If you are looking for serious day hiking or a place to camp prior to backpacking, Colorado Canyon provides the best access to more than 25 miles of true wilderness on the Rancherias Trail. There is also a river trail between Colorado Canyon and the other two tent campgrounds, Madera Canyon and Grassy Banks. These last two also allow trailers, but the lack of electricity and sewer hookups keep most RVs away.

Whatever your interest, this park will provide even the most rugged outdoor enthusiast in your group a significant physical challenge and solitary experience.

VOICES FROM THE CAMPFIRE AND RECOMMENDED READING

The Spanish explorers were lured by the tales of cities whose streets were paved with gold, and their imaginations were fired to such an extent that they were willing to endure almost unbelievable hardships to realize their dreams.

Ross A. Maxwell, *The Big Bend of the Rio Grande: A Guide to the Rocks, Landscape, Geologic History, and Settlers of the Area of Big Bend National Park* (Austin, University of Texas, 1968).

BACKCOUNTRY ADVENTURES

Some trails are designated for hikers only, but mountain bikers and horseback riders alike may enjoy other trails in this rugged and secluded area. Guided tours, trip options, and rental horses available from Lajitas Stables, the park's equestrian outfitter. Bring your own horse ($2/day, plus permit.)

BEST LOCAL FOOD AND DRINK

Give your boots or saddle a rest and mosey into The Enlightened Bean Café in Presidio (432-229-3131). Breakfasts are reported to really shine. Also good are the hamburgers, Mexican entrées, and more (BYOB.) Or experience the Starlight Theatre Restaurant & Saloon in Terlingua (432-371-3400; thestarlighttheatre.com). A onetime movie palace, this offbeat eatery offers innovative Texas eats and live music amid murals.

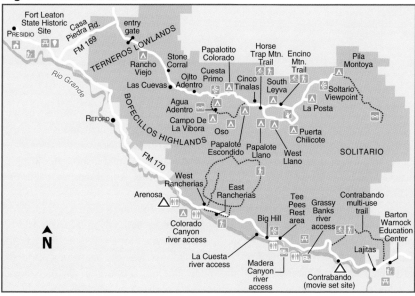

Big Bend Ranch State Park

GETTING THERE

From Presidio, travel 3 miles southeast on FM 170 to the Fort Leaton State Historic Site for registration, fee payment, and information about weather conditions and site availability.

From Lajitas and the ghost town of Terlingua, travel northwest on FM 170. The various sites are well marked along the road.

GPS COORDINATES:
FORT LEATON: N29° 32.551' W104° 19.581'
BARTON WARNOCK: N29° 16.194' W103° 45.441'

6

Davis Mountains State Park

Beauty: ★★★★ / Privacy: ★★★ / Spaciousness: ★★★ / Quiet: ★★★ / Security: ★★★★ / Cleanliness: ★★★★

Whichever tent site you choose, you will enjoy excellent shade trees and close proximity to Keesey Creek.

Named after historic Fort Davis, the Davis Mountains provide a perfect home for this state park and tent campers seeking relief from the heat and humidity of other Texas campgrounds. Located at more than 5,000 feet, the campground stretches along the mostly dry Keesey Creek and is sheltered by a mixture of mature pine, juniper, and oak trees as well as the neighboring volcanic peaks. This 2,700-acre park was developed between 1933 and 1935 by the Civilian Conservation Corps, whose stonework remains intact and symbolizes workers grateful for even backbreaking employment during the Great Depression. One of the best examples is the Indian Lodge, completed in 1935. Now fully restored, it continues to serve travelers escaping the lowland heat or traveling to other, more remote parts of this dry and beautiful country.

The tent-camping sites are located along Park Road 3 and begin just past the turnoff to RV sites 1–61. In order to select the best and most private tent-camping areas, continue on Park Road 3, passing sites 62–67 until the Indian Lodge appears on your right. Turn left and cross the low-water crossing of Keesey Creek to find sites 68–94, which will give you some excellent choices. Site 80, for example, is not only large but also has easy access to the bathroom and showers. Whichever tent site you choose, you will enjoy excellent shade trees and close proximity to Keesey Creek, which is dry most of the year, but do be cautious in heavy rainfall

Tent camping with a view

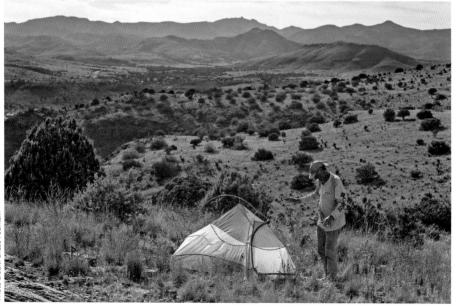

Photo credit: Chase Fountain

KEY INFORMATION

ADDRESS: TX 118 N, Fort Davis, TX 79734 (park is 3 miles northwest of Fort Davis, TX)

OPERATED BY: Texas Parks & Wildlife Department

CONTACT: 432-426-3337, tpwd.texas.gov /state-parks/davis-mountains

OPEN: Year-round

SITES: 94

EACH SITE: Picnic table, fire ring, water

ASSIGNMENT: First come, first served until site-specific reservation system begins in 2018

REGISTRATION: At entrance station or reserve at texas.reserveworld.com or 512-389-8900

FACILITIES: Clean, modern bathrooms

PARKING: At each site

FEE: $15/night for water-only campsites; $6/person entrance fee

ELEVATION: 5,038'

RESTRICTIONS:

PETS: On leash only

FIRES: Burn ban may be in effect. Contact park for update.

ALCOHOL: Prohibited in all public/ outdoor areas

VEHICLES: 2/site

OTHER: Maximum 8 people/site; guests must leave by 10 p.m.; quiet time 10 p.m.– 6 a.m.; bring your own charcoal; limited supplies available at park store, located at entrance station; pick up other supplies in Fort Davis; gathering firewood prohibited

conditions. The towering Davis Mountains and surrounding rocky terrain also shelter the campground, making for a wilderness experience in the high desert of West Texas.

While this campground appears quite civilized, the park advises you to beware of bears, mountain lions, and javelinas, and not to leave small children or pets unattended. It is also important to store your food inside a closed vehicle to prevent attracting wild animals to the campground.

Besides the mild climate of the Davis Mountains, the area also offers the vistas of Skyline Drive, which is within the park and overlooks the town of Fort Davis and the Fort Davis National Historic Site—a must-see. This frontier fort has a large number of buildings that have been expertly restored. The visitor center and museum offer a fascinating glimpse of Texas history and a chance to learn not only about American Indians who inhabited this area, but also the famous "buffalo soldiers" who were assigned to Fort Davis after the Civil War.

After leaving the state park, turn left on TX 118 and travel 14 miles to the internationally known McDonald Observatory, which has hosted astronomers since 1939. Its location on 6,791-foot Mt. Locke enjoys the darkest skies in the continental United States, and day and night tours are offered. While camping at Davis Mountains State Park, be sure to attend a Star Party to see heavenly sights a city dweller can only imagine.

VOICES FROM THE CAMPFIRE AND RECOMMENDED READING

As darkness falls, though, an even more spectacular canvas unfolds overhead. The dark sky begins to blaze with stars. . . . And when the Milky Way arcs overhead, it looks like a shimmering river of light.

(McDonald Observatory Guide, 2008)

Available at Fort Davis National Historic Site, *Black Frontiersman: The Memoirs of Henry O. Flipper* by Theodore D. Harris chronicles the first black graduate of West Point and his assignment to Fort Davis as one of the famous Buffalo Soldiers.

BACKCOUNTRY ADVENTURES

The park's new specially designed bird blind has become a favorite for viewing a multitude of common and elusive bird species, photographing, or just relaxing. Check the park's calendar for special interpretive programs and birding walks. A must-see attraction is the restored Fort Davis complex, where visitors can catch a glimpse of life on the Texas frontier.

BEST LOCAL FOOD AND DRINK

Locals and visitors alike enjoy Hebert's Caboose Ice Cream Shop (432-426-3141). For food, drink, and ice cream options, stop by the Fort Davis Drug Store (432-426-3929; fortdavis drugstore.net). Call for current/seasonal hours.

Davis Mountains State Park

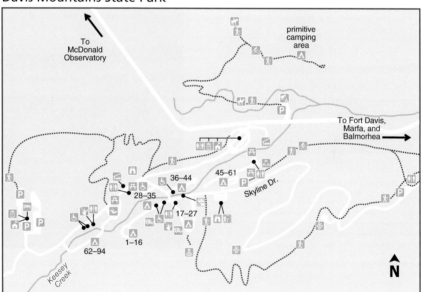

GETTING THERE

From Fort Davis, drive west 3 miles on TX 118. The park entrance will be on your left.

GPS COORDINATES: N30° 35.964' W103° 55.740'

7

Guadalupe Mountains National Park

Beauty: ★★★★★ / Privacy: ★★★ / Spaciousness: ★★★ / Quiet: ★★★★ / Security: ★★★★ / Cleanliness: ★★★★

Take the time to embrace the incredible mix of plant and animal life that thrives in this desert landscape.

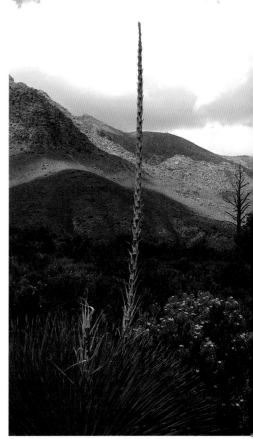

Reaching for the sky for a better view

Tent camping in the high desert is always a special experience. Add in the tallest mountain in Texas at 8,749 feet and surrounding sheer cliffs reaching 8,085 feet, and you have one of the premier tent-camping locales in the state. Guadalupe Mountains National Park, which opened in 1972, has 86,000 acres of wild terrain that invite discovery on foot or horseback. Like all deserts, the landscape here appears harsh and almost lifeless when viewed at high speed from an air-conditioned box, but taking the time to embrace the incredible mix of plant life and animals that thrive on the clear, clean, and surprisingly cool mountain air will bring ample rewards to those willing to slow down and stay awhile.

As you approach the park from either Van Horn or El Paso, the vast remoteness begins to sink in, and the first view of El Capitan's 2,000-foot-plus rock face brings easy comparisons to the more famous Yosemite Valley monolith. The Pine Springs Visitor Center turnoff is on your left and provides the best place to start your visit. There is an excellent small museum, and the rangers are glad to fill you in on the best hikes in the park and what conditions you will likely face in the backcountry. Note that the visitor center does not have supplies.

As with most national parks, you will need a backcountry permit for overnight stays, but day hikes are unrestricted. However, be sure to use the hiker's register at the trailhead so your absence might be noticed in a timelier manner should you stray, twist your ankle, or have an unscheduled meeting with a mountain lion or rattlesnake. Remember that 60% of this park has been designated official wilderness and must be respected as such.

Leaving the visitor center parking lot, Pine Springs Campground is on the right. The central parking lot contains the restrooms, marked RV spaces with no hookups, and the trailhead (which leads to the strenuous but spectacular 8.4-mile Guadalupe Peak Trail, where you can truly say you have been to the top of Texas).

KEY INFORMATION

ADDRESS: 400 Pine Springs to Guadalupe Peak, Salt Flat, Texas 79847

OPERATED BY: National Park Service

CONTACT: 915-828-3251, nps.gov/gumo; reservations: group sites only at 915-828-3251

OPEN: Year-round

SITES: 20 (Pine Springs Campground, 2 tent/6 people max); Group sites: 1 in Dog Canyon, 2 in Pine Springs

EACH SITE: Picnic table and level tent pad

ASSIGNMENT: First come, first served (group sites can be reserved up to 60 days in advance)

REGISTRATION: At registration station

FACILITIES: Modern restrooms with service sink but no showers; water

PARKING: At each site except 4–12

FEE: $5 entrance fee/7 days (annual pass $20); Campsites $8/site, $5/site with Golden Age Passport; $3/person at group site, $1.50/person with Golden Age Passport

ELEVATION: 5,707'

RESTRICTIONS:

PETS: On leash only; no pets on trails

FIRES: Prohibited but containerized fuel stoves allowed

ALCOHOL: Prohibited

VEHICLES: 1/site

OTHER: Maximum 2 tents/6 people/site; Group sites—minimum 10/maximum 20; guests must leave by 8 p.m.; quiet time 8 p.m.–8 a.m.; pick up supplies in El Paso, Van Horn, or Carlsbad; gathering firewood prohibited

Upon returning to the parking lot, the tent-camping road starts on your immediate left with sites 4–12 a short walk from the parking spots. The other sites each have one parking spot. All sites are nicely spaced, with level tent pads and unrestricted views of the Guadalupe Mountains, which not only draw the eye but also seem to beckon you to explore further. Two group sites are available for a minimum of 10 people or maximum of 20. If you are lucky enough to be here during a full moon, its fiery orange appearance on the eastern horizon will help you understand the reverence paid the moon by the Mescalero Apaches, who thrived here until the European explorers decided to convert them to their own religion and civilization, with or without their consent.

Leaving the tent-camping area, return to US 62/180 and turn left. Drive 0.3 mile and stop at the Pinery Butterfield Stage Ruins for a lesson on the real Old West. In 1858 this station acted as a true oasis for the passengers, drivers, and horses that were part of the first intercontinental mail route from St. Louis to San Francisco. The route was chosen to avoid the dangerous mountains to the north, but instead encroached on American Indian territory to the south. It only lasted until the Civil War, but it remains a true monument to courage and endurance prior to the era of railroads, which replaced the stagecoach on this long and dangerous route.

Continuing on the main highway, travel north just under 7 miles until you reach the McKittrick Canyon turnoff on your left. This day-use area contains another must-see Texas trail. The 6.8-mile round-trip McKittrick Canyon Trail leads you deep into the park and a rich landscape that mixes prickly pear cacti and agaves with a canyon woodland of willows, alligator junipers, ponderosa pines, and the most beautiful Texas madrones, whose trunk and limbs turn almost red alongside the smooth, tan bark. This trail is rated moderate for a rough surface, but the persistent hiker will be rewarded for the effort. In the fall, the foliage explodes into colors even a Northeasterner can appreciate.

A final stop will require a 2-hour drive north into New Mexico past Carlsbad Caverns National Park. From Pine Springs Visitor Center, take US 62E/US 180 E for 44.4 miles, then take a left onto Dark Canyon Road (CR 408) and drive about 22 miles. Take another left on NM 137 and drive 34.4 miles to Dog Canyon Campground. Here you'll find nine walk-in tent sites with drinking water, restrooms, and a ranger station. The elevation is 6,300 feet and will give you excellent access to the high country, including a secluded, forested canyon on this little-used north side of the park. Bring some good hiking boots and all your supplies to stay awhile in one of the least-known but truly wild tent-camping spots in Texas. Be sure to check on current availability of this campground, as flooding on NM 137 can close the road.

VOICES FROM THE CAMPFIRE AND RECOMMENDED READING

What draws us into the desert is the search for something intimate in the remote.
    Edward Abbey, *A Voice Crying in the Wilderness* (New York, St. Martin's Press, 1989).

I am not always in sympathy with nature-study as pursued in the schools, as if this kingdom could be carried by assault. Such study is too cold, too special, too mechanical; it is likely to rub the bloom off Nature. It lacks soul and emotions; it misses the accessories of the open air and its exhilarations, the sky, the clouds, the landscape, and the currents of life that pulse everywhere.
    John Burroughs, Chapter XIII: The Gospel of Nature, *The Writings of John Burroughs, Volume XIV: Time and Change* (Boston, Houghton Mifflin Company, 1912).

Your first view of El Capitan

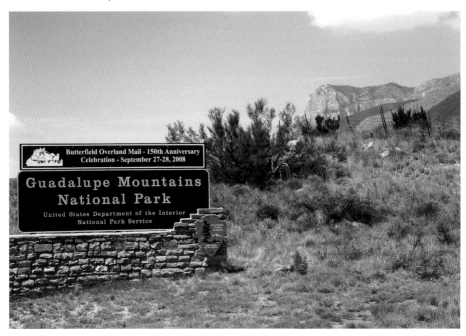

BACKCOUNTRY ADVENTURES

This wilderness park is full of opportunities to test the endurance of any intrepid explorer. The trek to Guadalupe Peak is a requirement for all able Texans who want to say they have climbed the highest peak in Texas. An equally beautiful trek is McKittrick Canyon in the fall. Check with park officials for the best equestrian trails, but bring your own horse, like any true Texan should. On your way back to El Paso, stop in to Hueco Tanks State Park for not only nice tent-camping sites but also rock climbing. For information, contact Albert Alvarez at Sessions Climbing (915-443-0340; sessionsclimbing.com).

BEST LOCAL FOOD AND DRINK

The park has little more than water to offer in the way of supplies. Be sure to stop in Van Horn, Texas, or White City, New Mexico, for a last chance meal and gas. Van Horn locals enjoy the dining and restored hotel charm of the El Capitan (877-283-1220; thehotelelcapitan.com) and breakfast and lunch at the Country Bagel (432-283-7262; countrybagel.net).

Guadalupe Mountains National Park

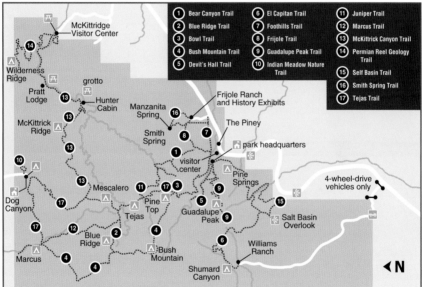

GETTING THERE

From El Paso, take US 62 E/US 180 E about 96 miles, then turn left at Pine Canyon Dr. and follow signs for the campground.

From Carlsbad, NM, take US 62 W/US 180 W about 53 miles, then turn right onto Pine Canyon Dr. and follow signs for the campground.

Please see the profile for directions to Dog Canyon Campground from Pine Springs Visitor Center.

GPS COORDINATES: N31° 50.364' W104° 49.860'

CENTRAL TEXAS AND THE HILL COUNTRY

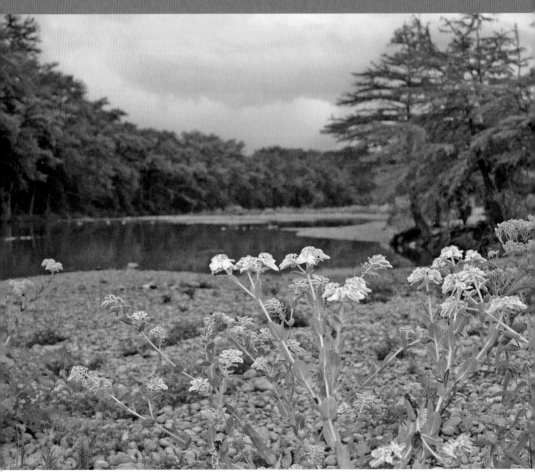

Springtime in Garner State Park (see page 48)

8

Bastrop and Buescher State Parks

Beauty: ★★★★ / Privacy: ★★★ / Spaciousness: ★★★ / Quiet: ★★★ / Security: ★★★★ / Cleanliness: ★★★

Slow down and enjoy this unique island of towering piney woods, now rising from the ashes.

Leaving the historic town of Bastrop on TX 21, Bastrop State Park has a rugged side and a history worthy of a Texas legend. Over the last century, this park has seen the apparent destruction of nature's beauty by clear-cutting and then wildfires, which blackened the sky with smoke and flames. These raging fires also threatened the dining hall, swimming area, and historic cabins completed by the Civilian Conservation Corps (CCC) in the 1930s. During this time, these young men not only built structures, roads, and campground areas, but they also seeded and transplanted a new forest of loblolly pines to repair the overused land. By a stroke of good luck, when the wildfire of 1942 struck, workers from CCC camps at Lake Austin and Seguin were still in the area and arrived in time to save the now historic structures and much of the forest from the flames. From this near miss forward, the park continued to increase in popularity including a National Historic Landmark designation and trees growing tall and thick enough to resemble the piney woods of East Texas located more than 100 miles away. These Lost Pines became a true arboreal island that gave campers and hikers a place to relax in shade.

In 2011 and 2015, this park was again struck by raging and life-threatening wildfires of sufficient magnitude to destroy the park structures and the ecosystem to a point where the Lost Pines might have been truly lost. However, just like the brave CCC companies of 1942, a combined massive effort of equally brave and determined firefighters eventually got the flames under control and saved the structures along with part of the forest. To all of these people, all lovers of the land owe a huge debt of gratitude.

After these two fires, the park is truly rising from the ashes to repair camping areas and hiking trails, but most important, the trees are being replanted and just like the fires of Yellowstone and many other great Western parks, the natural beauty is returning with incredible speed. While these fires are always terrifying, the burned areas now provide life-giving nutrients to the soil and additional sunlight to the understory.

Just like the clear-cutters could not destroy this special part of Texas, the fires will do nature's cleanup work and Bastrop State Park will return to its towering beauty and solace.

Bastrop State Park is a changed but still family-friendly destination with a surprisingly rugged side. The fires changed the landscape, and flooding in 2015 led to dam failure and more damage. Some areas of the park are closed due to the flood and fire damage and/or projects to repair them, and because of the dam failure, the park's 10-acre lake is gone. But there is still much to enjoy. Trails inside the Park Road 1A loop are open. As of publication date, the primitive camping and group youth areas are closed indefinitely. Check the park website or office for updates on the status of park roads and trails.

As you enter the park, the old golf course along the road is no longer part of your approach, but enough of the towering loblolly pines in this central Texas location survived the fires to invite you in. In place of the golf course, you'll see Lake Mina, a kid-friendly, 0.5-acre fishing hole. Leaving the entrance station on Park Road 1A, the dining hall and swimming area are 0.3 mile straight ahead. This CCC-built area is a National Historic Landmark and includes a large outdoor stone deck with smokers and grills for group reservations.

KEY INFORMATION

ADDRESS: Bastrop: 100 Park Road 1A, Bastrop, TX 78602
Buescher: 100 Park Road 1C, Smithville, TX 78957

CONTACT: 512-321-2101, tpwd.texas.gov /state-parks/bastrop (Bastrop); 512-237-2241, tpwd.texas.gov/state-parks /buescher (Buescher)

OPERATED BY: Texas Parks & Wildlife Department

OPEN: Year-round

SITES: Bastrop: 6 in Creekside, 16 in Deer Run, 19 in Copperas Creek. Buescher: 20 in Lakeview (drive up), 5 walk-in by reservation on site only

EACH SITE: Picnic table, fire ring, lantern hook

ASSIGNMENT: First come, first served until site-specific reservation system begins in 2018

REGISTRATION: At headquarters or reserve at texas.reserveworld.com or 512-389-8900

FACILITIES: Restrooms, showers in RV area, swimming pool, park store, dining hall for groups

PARKING: At each site except Copperas Creek

FEE: $12 water only; $10 primitive site; $5/person entrance fee

ELEVATION: 581'

RESTRICTIONS:
PETS: On leash only

FIRES: In fire rings

ALCOHOL: Prohibited in all public/ outdoor areas

VEHICLES: 2/site

OTHER: Maximum 8 people/site; guests must leave by 10 p.m.; quiet time 10 p.m.– 6 a.m.; bring your own firewood or charcoal; limited supplies at park store; pick up main supplies in Bastrop; gathering firewood prohibited

Turn left and then an immediate right toward campsites 1–42. Make another hard right into the day-use area or you will end up in the Piney Hill RV area. Back in the day-use area, the Deer Run Camping Area is past the playground and down a slight hill off a gravel road. Sites 36–42 are on the immediate right. Sites 31–35 are in the circular drive area and provide the most privacy for tent campers, but still provide easy access to the modern restrooms and showers. The sites all back up to a heavily wooded area shaded by the towering Lost Pines Forest.

As you venture out into the park, you begin to feel like you have taken a trip to Deep East Texas, even though you are 100 miles away from the similar Piney Woods region. This island of approximately 75,000 acres has persisted in the area for more than 18,000 years and has adapted to 30% less rainfall than its eastern Texas cousin. The park contains more than 11 miles of trails, including the Lost Pines Trail—which has multiple elevation changes and, when open, allows primitive camping with a permit for the backpackers in your group. For the less adventurous, a set of 12 historic cabins are located at the end of Park Road 1B. Even if you aren't staying in the cabins, visit this area for the rustic architecture.

Returning to the dining hall and swimming area, follow Park Road 1A to the Creekside Camping Area for walk-in sites 43–48. These primitive sites flank the 1.14-mile Scenic Overlook Trail and can also be accessed through the Copperas Creek RV Camping Area.

Whatever your interest—camping under the Lost Pines, hiking the challenging trail system, or just cruising scenic Park Road 1C to nearby Buescher State Park—Bastrop State Park is not to be missed.

As you leave Bastrop State Park on Park Road 1C, this little-known parkway will remind you of an earlier time when the CCC was busy building the infrastructure of our nation's national parks. The road's steep grades will deter most RVs. It is a popular bicycle path, so be sure to share the road. These hilly 7.5 miles are shaded by a wide variety of oaks and those Lost Pines, and contain some low-water crossings and a viewpoint to the right off a ridgeline.

As you reach the end of this Texas version of the Natchez Trace, the road dead-ends at the Lakeview Camping Area of Buescher State Park and sites 41–55. These nicely spaced sites start on the right and back up to a small creek area with huge moss-covered trees that provide much-needed summer shade. As you reach the circle and sites 46–49, you can see the 25-acre park lake and enjoy a small campground without the RV traffic. The tent sites are level and make an excellent base camp for bicycle trips or day hikes on the 7.7-mile Buescher Hiking Trail.

After site 49, look for the easy trail to walk-in sites 56–60 on the right. These well-hidden sites are just far enough off the road for campers to feel they have reached the wilderness without the exertion of carrying a backpack. Central parking and the main pavilion are on the left along with modern restrooms and showers just ahead on the right. Returning to Park Road 1E, turn right up the hill to find the Buescher Hiking trailhead and parking for walk-in sites 61–65. These sites off the road are easily accessible, and campers won't find an RV in sight. If you get lost and end up in the Cozy Circle Camping Area, you will find a no-tents sign. I guess not so cozy for everyone.

Whichever tent site you do choose, this Post Oak Savannah Ecoregion allows exploration of not only the famous Lost Pines, but also of endangered species, such as the Houston toad. There are also pileated woodpeckers here darting from tree to tree in their search for lunch or a nesting site.

Historic cabin saved by incredible bravery

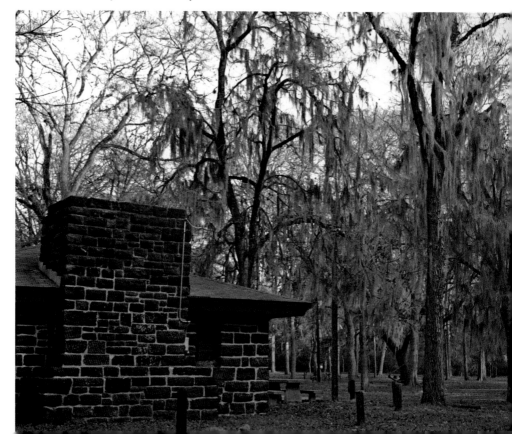

VOICES FROM THE CAMPFIRE AND RECOMMENDED READING

Bastrop—An erratic, persistent forest and brush fire, which spread over some 30,000 acres, was extinguished Thursday, after CCC-trained fire fighters had battled the conflagration for three to four days.

Cynthia Brandimarte with Angela Reed, Texas State Parks and the CCC: The Legacy of the Civilian Conservation Corps (College Station, Texas A&M University Press, 2013).

Author's note: Reported in area newspapers, March 12, 1942. The firefighters were from CCC camps in Lake Austin and Seguin.

Perhaps the last word should be given to Todd McClanahan, regional director and superintendent of Bastrop and Buescher State Parks: With the recent wildfires at Bastrop State Park, I've learned to appreciate these historic structures even more. Knowing just how close we came to losing them forever forces me to admire their beauty with a different perspective. They are so much more than historic buildings; they are historic treasures, which I hope someday my two sons will visit and reflect back on the days of their youth when they lived and played in two of the most important state parks in Texas.

Brandimarte with Reed, Texas State Parks and the CCC (2013).

BACKCOUNTRY ADVENTURES

While the fire has temporarily changed the landscape, the road between Bastrop and Buescher remains an excellent workout with ridgetop views. Another rewarding activity is to volunteer in the replanting of trees and nurturing this beautiful park back to health. You can easily feel the memories and presence of the CCC workers from the Depression. You are both helping make the future.

BEST LOCAL FOOD AND DRINK

Locals and campers alike enjoy a good burger and cold beer at the Roadhouse (512-321-1803; roadhousebastrop.com), just across from the entrance to Bastrop. For fried catfish or fried shrimp, pull into Paw-Paws Catfish House in Bastrop (512-321-9800; pawpawscatfish house.com), just a few miles away.

GETTING THERE

Bastrop: From the intersection of TX 71 and I-35 in Austin, take TX 71 W for 28.4 miles. Follow signs for TX 21 E/TX 95N and drive only 0.4 mile, then turn right onto TX 21 E/Chestnut St. and drive 0.8 mile. Turn right onto Park Road 1 and then left into the park entrance.

Buescher: From Bastrop State Park, take Park Road 1C from the eastern edge of Bastrop roughly 3 miles to the Lakeview Campground. From TX 71, travel 2 miles north on FM 153 to Park Road 1 and the Buescher entrance station.

GPS COORDINATES:
BASTROP: N30° 6.610' W97° 17.212'
BUESCHER: N30° 2.346' W97° 9.498'

Bastrop State Park

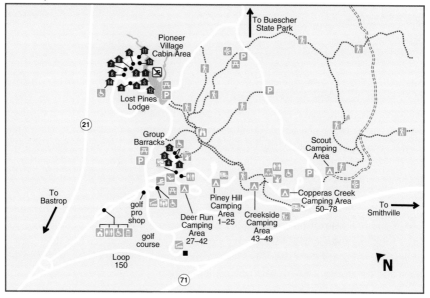

Buescher State Park

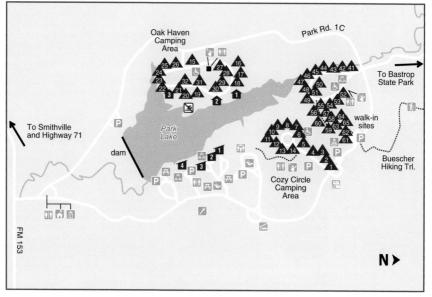

9

Colorado Bend State Park

Beauty: ★★★ / Privacy: ★★★ / Spaciousness: ★★★★ / Quiet: ★★★★ / Security: ★★★★ / Cleanliness: ★★★

Be sure to visit the spring-fed waterfall in this spectacular Hill Country setting.

If you are looking for remote beauty and a rare opportunity to camp next to a major river, then Colorado Bend State Park is a great destination. Leaving Llano on TX 16, you travel north 18.4 miles on one of the most scenic roads in Texas into the small town of Cherokee. Turn east (right) on Ranch Road 501 and follow the winding road until it dead-ends into FM 580. Turn right and follow the Colorado River until the road turns into County Road 436 at Bad Bob's Bend Store. Pick up last-minute supplies and proceed to this under-visited tent camper's paradise. The road has several low-water crossings with rangeland on both sides. The old gravel road is now smooth blacktop, but the surroundings over the next 10 or so miles will make you feel off the beaten path. Watch for deer and enjoy the rough terrain of cactus and rocks until you pass the park boundary. You'll see the Windmill Trail on your right at 1.2 miles and a great Hill Country view at 4.5 miles, just prior to a steep descent to park headquarters and the Colorado River. Check in with the park rangers at this remote outpost and get assistance with your campsite selection.

Gorman Falls is a hidden treasure.

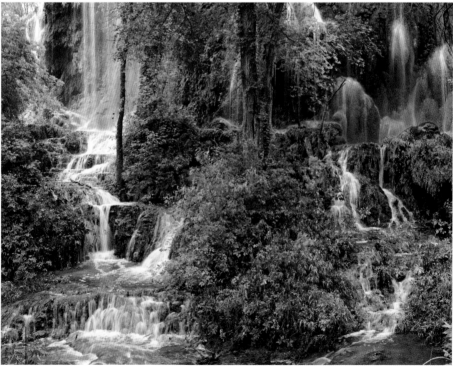

Photo credit: *Chase Fountain*

KEY INFORMATION

ADDRESS: 2236 Park Hill Dr., Bend, TX 76824

CONTACT: 800-792-1112 or 325-628-3240, tpwd.texas.gov/state-parks/colorado-bend

OPERATED BY: Texas Parks & Wildlife Department

OPEN: Year-round

SITES: 38 (drive up or walk in), 3 group sites (16, 25, and 48 people max, respectively)

EACH SITE: Central water, picnic table, fire pit, lantern hook

ASSIGNMENT: First come, first served until site-specific reservation system begins in 2018

REGISTRATION: At headquarters or reserve at texas.reserveworld.com or 512-389-8900

FACILITIES: Park store, chemical toilets, kayak rentals

PARKING: At each site; short walk to riverside sites

FEE: $13 riverside walk-in sites; $15 drive-up sites; three group sites: $25/$40/$75; $5/person entrance fee, age 12 and under free

ELEVATION: 1,069'

RESTRICTIONS:

PETS: On leash only

FIRES: In fire pits

ALCOHOL: Prohibited in all public/outdoor areas

VEHICLES: 2/site

OTHER: Maximum 8 people/site; guests must leave by 10 p.m.; quiet time 10 p.m.– 6 a.m.; bring your own firewood or charcoal; limited supplies at park store; pick up main supplies in Llano or San Saba

The park's campsites were renumbered a few years ago. Sites 1–16 are to your right and numbered parking spaces are to your left. The campsites are down a small embankment and spread on a large grassy knoll next to the Colorado River. Look for riverside site 1 under a large clump of willow trees, or site 2 under a huge pecan tree. All these sites have river views, and a massive rock wall on the other side hides the campground from the outside world.

Continue on the main park road toward the group campground and day-use area. Look for the Spicewood Springs trailhead at the end of the parking lot and follow the tree-lined path to a series of small pools and waterfalls as they cascade down the hillside. The trail also heads uphill, and at the top, you leave the "tourist" area and start into some real wilderness. Watch for Texas-size red ants and silver dollar–size spiders that seem to like to spin their symmetrical webs between the junipers and directly across the trail. Luckily, it's easy to go around these scary-looking friends, but don't forget to check the trail ahead for the far-more dangerous diamondback rattlesnakes as they wait in the shade or come out in the cool of the evening after the hot Texas sun heads toward the horizon.

If you happen upon any of these vipers, give them a wide berth and head quickly back to the campground and peaceful riverside sites 18–25. Sites 40 and 41 are near the composting toilet, and Site 26 is a large, private site near enough to hear the river. Sites 35–39 are away from the river, but have the protection of a rock escarpment and nice tree cover. They also allow close-in parking.

As you enjoy the camping, don't miss the chance to rent kayaks or take the ranger-guided tour to Gorman Falls. The $5-per-person cost is well worth the chance to see a spring-fed waterfall in a spectacular Hill Country setting. It's a 1.5-mile round-trip walk, so bring your water and camera for a special treat to finish off your visit to this remote location. The hike is mostly flat but has a surprisingly steep, but short incline just before you reach the riverbed area. Chains along the rock help ease your descent/ascent. Whether you're with a ranger or on your own, don't miss this scenic gem! For those adventurous souls without fear of tight spaces, there is weekend access to Wild Cave and Gorman Cave, but be sure to make reservations (online only) with Nichols Outdoor Adventures at cbcaves.com.

VOICES FROM THE CAMPFIRE AND RECOMMENDED READING

We are now ready to start on our way down the Great Unknown. . . . We have an unknown distance yet to run; an unknown river yet to explore. What falls there are, we know not; what rocks beset the channel, we know not; what walls rise over the river, we know not.

John Wesley Powell, Exploration of the Colorado River of the West and Its Tributaries (Washington, Government Printing Office, 1875).

Author's note: Written on August 13, 1869, as Powell entered the Grand Canyon.

BACKCOUNTRY ADVENTURES

The numerous hiking trails are excellent opportunities to get away from the crowds. This remote park has not only Spicewood Springs and Gorman Falls to enjoy, but also enough arid and cactus-covered country to remind you that you are still in Texas.

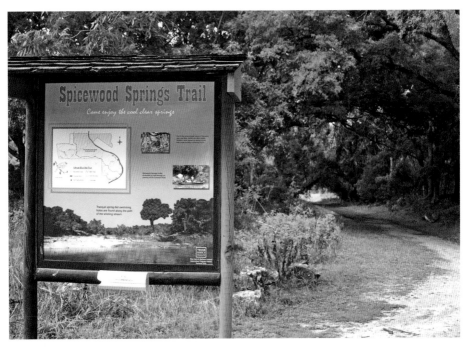

The Spicewood Springs Trail starts out easy but ends in the wild backcountry.

BEST LOCAL FOOD AND DRINK

Bad Bob's Bend Store (325-628-3523) no longer offers grilled hamburgers but is still the closest place for ice cream, snacks, simple grocery items, and supplies. If you crave a great hamburger, drive to Lampasas, where folks have been pulling into Storm's Drive-In (512-556-6269; stormsrestaurants.com) since 1950 or Eva's Cafe on the Square (512-556-3500; evesonthesquare.com) for awesome German dishes. Cooper's Old Time Pit BBQ in Llano (325-247-5713; coopersbbqllano.com) would also be a treat after a day of hiking. Both towns are about a 30-minute drive from the park entrance.

Colorado Bend State Park

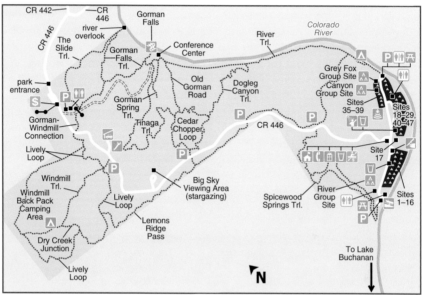

GETTING THERE

From San Saba, travel east 3.5 miles on US 190. Turn right (south) onto FM 580 and drive 14 miles to Bend. Continue onto County Road 442 and drive 0.8 mile, then turn right to stay on CR 442. After another 2.2 miles, turn right onto CR 446, and in 0.6 mile you'll reach the park entrance.

GPS COORDINATES: N31° 1.350' W98° 26.550'

10

Enchanted Rock State Natural Area

Beauty: ★★★★ / Privacy: ★★★★ / Spaciousness: ★★★★ / Quiet: ★★★★ / Security: ★★★★ / Cleanliness: ★★★

The huge slickrock dome will have you wondering if a wrong turn didn't land you in the canyon lands of Utah.

As you approach Enchanted Rock State Natural Area on Ranch Road 965, the huge slickrock dome and surrounding formations will have you checking your map to see if a wrong turn didn't land you in the canyon lands of Utah. In fact, your first view of the park area will remind you of the eastern approach to Zion National Park.

As you pass the entrance station and enter the park, the RVs and trailers are diverted into a parking lot on the left, while the tent campers and day hikers cross over a wide low-water crossing into the main camping area. Continuing to the right toward the day-use area, the parking for sites 35–46 is on your left. These sites are a short walk into the trees toward Enchanted Rock and will give you excellent access to the summit trail.

Returning back toward the low-water crossing, the modern bathrooms and showers are on your left, along with tent sites 4–20. These nicely spaced sites are set back from the road for a little extra quiet. Sites 17, 19, and 21 are the most private and back up to Sandy Creek. These sites also provide an excellent vantage point to view Enchanted Rock and the surrounding rugged landscape.

Visit this park when the tourists go home.

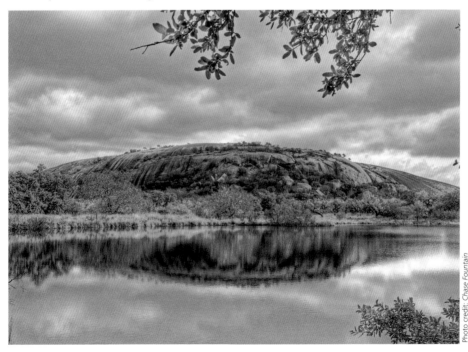

Photo credit: *Chase Fountain*

KEY INFORMATION

ADDRESS: 16710 Ranch Road 965,
Fredericksburg, TX 78624

OPERATED BY: Texas Parks & Wildlife
Department

CONTACT: 830-685-3636,
tpwd.texas.gov/state-parks/enchanted-rock

OPEN: Year-round

SITES: 35 walk-in sites, 1 group site
(private entrance, must hike in 1.5 mile)

EACH SITE: Picnic table, fire pit, lantern
hook; the park requests that you bring
your own water, as it is in short supply due
to drought

ASSIGNMENT: First come, first served
until site-specific reservation system
begins in 2018

REGISTRATION: At entrance station/
headquarters or reserve at
texas.reserveworld.com or 512-389-8900

FACILITIES: Centrally located modern
restrooms and showers

PARKING: Central lots

FEE: $18/walk-in tent site with water;
$100 private group camping area;
$7/adult entrance fee, $3 age 65 and
older, age 12 and under free

ELEVATION: 1,389'

RESTRICTIONS:

PETS: On leash only on loop trail, not upper
trails, must be personally attended in
campsites

FIRES: In fire pits

ALCOHOL: Prohibited

VEHICLES: 2/site

OTHER: Maximum 8 people/individual site,
75 max at group site; guests must leave by
10 p.m.; quiet time 10 p.m.–6 a.m.; bring
your own firewood or charcoal; limited
supplies at park store; fill gas tank and pick
up main supplies in Fredericksburg or
Llano; gathering firewood prohibited

Returning to the parking area, the other side of the road will allow close-in access to some of the premier campsites in Texas. A short walk across wooden bridges will lead you into a heavily wooded area and site numbers 23 and higher. These sites are well spaced and divided by underbrush and rocky ravines. The white-tailed deer scurry between the tents, and you'll immediately feel a sense of peacefulness. There is also a sense of grandeur looming just a few feet away as these sites nestle close to the smooth sandstone monolith that makes this park a popular stop for all Texas travelers visiting the Hill Country. This destination is so popular that weekends are not only totally booked with campers, but the park has been forced to limit the number of additional cars with day-use hikers, picnickers, or those just pondering the view. Get there early, go during the week, or pick the worst weather day you can visit. Maybe not a Texas tornado or flash flood kind of day, but a really cold day in the hill country is a true breath of fresh air.

After you pitch your tent, put on hiking boots or good sturdy tennis shoes and head to the Summit trailhead located at the end of the day-use parking lot. This short 0.6-mile trail climbs a steep 425 feet but is well worth the effort. Be sure not to hurry, but enjoy the panoramic views along with the hearty cactus and juniper appearing to grow out of solid rock. Take plenty of water and a bit of food so you can stay and ponder the beauty laid out before you.

Returning to the campground, the Loop Trail is a very nice 4-mile walk that will take you around the rock and to the primitive camping areas. There are also excellent opportunities to practice your rock-climbing skills, but registration with park headquarters is required.

As you leave the park, allow sufficient time to enjoy Fredericksburg, one of Texas's great Hill Country towns. The main street is lined with historic storefronts. The National

Museum of the Pacific War has been updated and expanded to truly honor native Texan Admiral Chester Nimitz.

The other famous attraction that cannot be missed is the spring wildflower season. Perennial Texas natives, including multicolored bluebonnets, Indian paintbrush, and Indian blanket cover roadsides and field after field. Mix in the flowering cactus and the awesome sight of Enchanted Rock and you quickly understand the irresistible lure of the Texas Hill Country.

VOICES FROM THE CAMPFIRE AND RECOMMENDED READING

Tell me what you will of the benefactions of city civilization. . . . I know that our bodies were made to thrive only in pure air, and the scenes in which pure air is found. If the death exhalations that brood the broad towns in which we so fondly compact ourselves were made visible, we should flee as from a plague.

John Muir, *John of the Mountains: The Unpublished Journals of John Muir* (Madison, University of Wisconsin Press, 1979).

From the summit were seen in unrivalled combination all the views which had rejoiced our eyes during the ascent. It was something at last to stand upon the storm-rent crown of this lonely sentinel of the Rocky Range, on one of the mightiest of the vertebrae of the backbone of the North American continent, and to see the waters start for both oceans. Uplifted above love and hate and storms of passion, calm amidst the eternal silences fanned by zephyrs and bathed in living blue, peace rested for that one bright day on the Peak.

Ann Ronald, ed., "Isabella Bird," Words for the Wild: The Sierra Club Trailside Reader (San Francisco, Sierra Club, 1987).

BACKCOUNTRY ADVENTURES

Take the hike around Enchanted Rock to get a full sense of its size and grandeur. It will leave 99% of the other park visitors behind in about 5 minutes. The primitive sites are good for beginner backpacking trips for those just getting started. Another place to visit is the Old Tunnel State Park, south of Fredericksburg, where between May and October you can witness up to 3 million Mexican free-tailed bats pouring into the sky for a nightly meal of mosquitos and other edibles. West of Enchanted Rock, toward Junction, Texas, is South Llano River State Park, which has added 2,200 acres of wildlife management area to its already popular river activities, including kayaking and canoeing. There is tent camping, but the river's pristine and cool water mean that reservations are always recommended.

BEST LOCAL FOOD AND DRINK

If you're up for a short drive, take the road south to Fredericksburg, where you'll find a myriad of restaurants, including Alamo Springs General Store (830-990-8004) or Burger Burger (830-997-5226; burgerburgerfbg.com) for, yes, a great burger, Cranky Frank's (830-997-2353; crankyfranksbbq.com) for finger-licking-good barbecue, Old German Bakery and Restaurant (830-997-9084; oldgermanbakeryandrestaurant.com) for German fare and breads, and the Cabernet Grill Texas Wine Country Restaurant (830-990-5734; cabernetgrill.com) or Fredericksburg Brewery Co. (844-596-2303; yourbrewery.com) for a liquid treat with good food.

Enchanted Rock State Natural Area

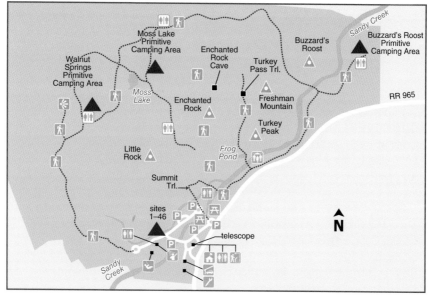

GETTING THERE

From Fredericksburg, go north on Ranch Road 965 for 17 miles. The park entrance is on your left.

GPS COORDINATES: N30° 29.748' W98° 49.218'

This low-water crossing leaves the RVs behind.

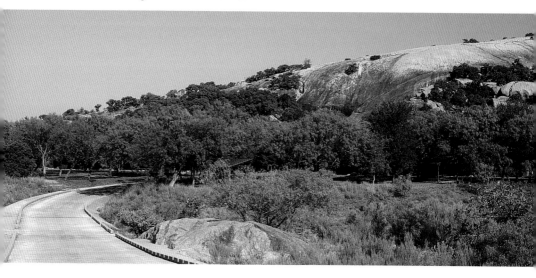

11

Garner State Park

Beauty: ★★★★ / Privacy: ★★★ / Spaciousness: ★★★ / Quiet: ★★★ / Security: ★★★ / Cleanliness: ★★★

This spring-fed river provides a genuine oasis to Texans looking for summer relief.

You can tell a park is popular when the drive up to the entrance station has traffic lanes similar to a sports arena or a large amusement park. There is also a radio frequency for current information about this rather remote but special place. As you enter the park, be sure to get the extensive and detailed map to assist you in finding your campsite and begin exploring why Garner State Park has such a high number of visitors.

After leaving the entrance station, proceed 0.5 mile and turn left at the intersection toward Persimmon Hill Camping Area and sites 200–234. These sites enjoy adequate tree cover, and even-numbered sites 200–214 on your right back up to a steep cliff and your first views of the Rio Frio. This spring-fed river flows gently through the rolling terrain of the Texas Hill Country and provides a genuine oasis to Texans looking for summer relief. As the name of the river aptly describes, the water is wonderfully cool even on the hottest afternoon. Look for sites 204 and 210 to have the best river views, but do be careful of the cliff if out wandering at night. As an added bonus, there are central bathrooms with showers for the Persimmon Hill tent campers.

Returning to the main road, proceed past the Live Oak RV area, and turn left into the Rio Frio Camping Area. Stay to the left after passing the sand volleyball court and continue

Cool water on a hot summer day is a true Texas surprise.

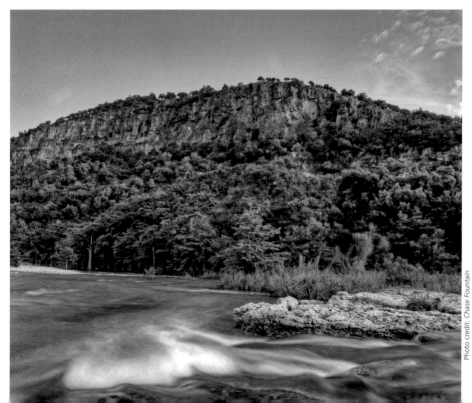

Photo credit: Chase Fountain

KEY INFORMATION

ADDRESS: 234 RR 1050, Concan, TX 78838

CONTACT: 800-792-1112 or 830-232-6132, tpwd.texas.gov/state-parks/garner

OPERATED BY: Texas Parks & Wildlife Department

OPEN: Year-round

SITES: 49 at Pecan Grove (Old Garner), 34 at Persimmon Hill, and 41 at Rio Frio (New Garner)

EACH SITE: Picnic table, fire ring, lantern hook, water

ASSIGNMENT: First come, first served until site-specific reservation system begins in 2018

REGISTRATION: At headquarters or reserve at texas.reserveworld.com or 512-389-8900

FACILITIES: Modern bathrooms and showers, visitor center, sand volleyball courts, trails

PARKING: At each site

FEE: $15–$20/night depending on location and date; $8/person entrance fee

ELEVATION: 1,413'

RESTRICTIONS:

PETS: On leash only

FIRES: In fire rings

ALCOHOL: Prohibited in all public/outdoor areas

VEHICLES: 2/site

OTHER: Maximum 8 people/site; guests must leave by 10 p.m.; quiet time 10 p.m.–6 a.m.; bring your own firewood or charcoal; limited supplies at park store or Leakey; pick up main supplies in Uvalde or Utopia

---

down the hill to sites 467–444. There is parking at each site and the river is on your left about 50 yards away. The river is obscured by heavy brush, but numerous trails lead through the sand dunes to the gently flowing water. On a quiet night, or while enjoying an early cup of tea or coffee, you can hear the flowing ripples. You can also hear the rumble of nearby thunderstorms, which is a reminder to heed any warnings from the park rangers. While the spring-fed water's level is fairly constant, heavy rainfall upstream can send this serene river into a massive flash flood that will clean and rearrange the sandbars for the next visitors.

At the river, you will find not only sandy beaches and gentle wading areas but also deep swimming holes and towering cypress trees with ropes to swing out on. Even if you are not climbing the big trees for a high dive, just watching Garner's visitors will conjure up an earlier time when going swimming, for generations of Americans, meant a lake, a river, or an ocean.

Returning to the main road, go past the River Crossing Camp Area and follow the signs to the day-use area and the pavilion. This drive will take you back up the hill for a great view of the entire park. As you descend, the Pecan Grove Camping Area is straight ahead, with some 49 water-only sites. They are shaded by huge pecan trees and are close to the most popular day-use areas, including swimming and paddleboats. These sites are good for families wishing to stay close to activities, but probably a little too busy for tent campers seeking solitude. Continuing past the day-use area, the pavilion is on your right. The Civilian Conservation Corps constructed this fine stone structure between 1935 and 1941. It contains a large dance floor and continues to host entertainment for all ages during the year.

As you enjoy the park's 9 miles of hiking trails, watch for the native white-tailed deer, Rio Grande turkeys, and even endangered species such as the golden-cheeked warbler and the black-capped vireo. You also might see an occasional Texas jackrabbit, just to remind you where you are and the harsh environment that surrounds this true oasis in the hills.

VOICES FROM THE CAMPFIRE AND RECOMMENDED READING

It was the cool gray dawn, and there was a delicious sense of repose and peace in the deep pervading calm and silence of the woods. Not a leaf stirred; not a sound obtruded upon great Nature's meditation.

Mark Twain, *The Adventures of Tom Sawyer* (Hartford, CT, American Publishing Co., 1876).

BACKCOUNTRY ADVENTURES

If the weekend summer crowds at Garner are too much, head north toward Vanderpool and Lost Maples State Natural Area. This area is famous for its fall color, so expect crowds then, but the rest of the year presents a wide range of hiking trails and a nice tent-camping area.

BEST LOCAL FOOD AND DRINK

For a breakfast taco or sandwich within the park, head to the Garner Grill. For local favorites north of the park, head into Leakey for a variety of good choices, including Mexican dishes at Mama Chole's (830-232-6111) or a full menu and buffet at Mill Creek Cafe (830-232-4805; millcreekcafeleakey.com).

Garner State Park

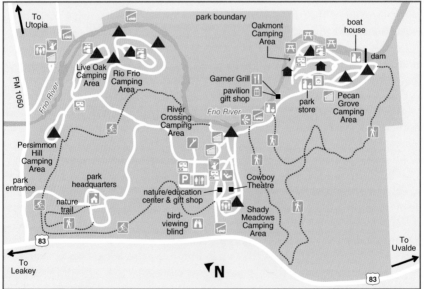

GETTING THERE

From US 90 in Uvalde, take US 83 north 31 miles to FM 1050. Turn right and drive 2 miles to Park Road 29. Turn right into the park.

GPS COORDINATES: N29° 35.952' W99° 44.598'

12

⚠ Guadalupe River State Park

Beauty: ★★★★ / Privacy: ★★★ / Spaciousness: ★★★ / Quiet: ★★★ / Security: ★★★ / Cleanliness: ★★★

Wagon Ford Walk-In Tent Area provides some of the best tent camping you will find.

Located only 30 miles north of San Antonio and 13 miles east of Boerne, this popular and scenic park is a must-stay camping stop. Be sure to start your wilderness adventure by picking up vital supplies at the Bear Moon Bakery and Cafe (830-816-2327; bearmoonbakery.com) in historic downtown Boerne. Once you're loaded with enough pastries and baked goods for the weekend, travel east on TX 46, turning north on Park Road 31 for 3.2 miles to the park head-quarters, where the friendly rangers will assist you in selecting the best available site.

At 1.3 miles, stop at the entrance to the Honey Creek State Natural Area. Guided tours are the only access to this pristine watershed. Scheduled at 9 a.m. on Saturdays, these tours take you into a fragile ecosystem of centuries-old cypress trees, ancient oaks, pecans, wal-nuts, cedar elms, and ash juniper trees, where the endangered golden-cheeked warbler finds a sheltered habitat.

Continuing on the main road for 0.1 mile, turn left into Cedar Sage Camping Area, sites 1–37. Your first right turn will take you to sites 6–13, which have nice spacing and tree cover. Sites 6, 8, and 9 back up to a heavily wooded canyon for a little wilderness feel and extra privacy. Sites 1–5 are along the road but are well spaced. Traveling toward the back

Visit this park's popular day-use area on a weekday to avoid the crowds.

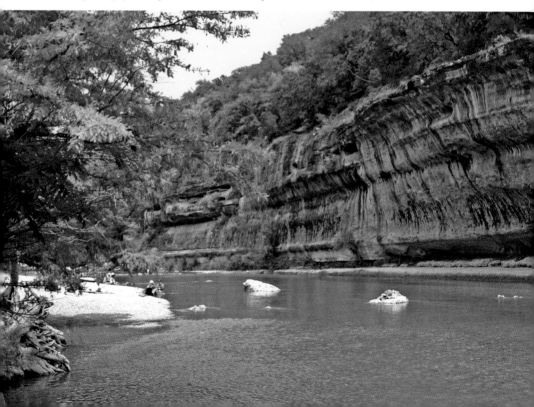

KEY INFORMATION

ADDRESS: 3350 Park Road 31,
Spring Branch, TX 78070

CONTACT: 830-438-2656,
tpwd.texas.gov/state-parks/guadalupe-river

OPERATED BY: Texas Parks & Wildlife Dept.

OPEN: Year-round

SITES: 37 in Cedar Sage, 9 in Wagon Ford

EACH SITE: Picnic table, fire ring,
lantern hook

ASSIGNMENT: First come, first served
until site-specific reservation system
begins in 2018

REGISTRATION: At headquarters or reserve
at texas.reserveworld.com or
512-389-8900

FACILITIES: Modern restrooms and showers
at Cedar Sage, restrooms at Wagon Ford

PARKING: At each site in Cedar Ridge;
central parking at Wagon Ford

FEE: $15–$20/night; $7/person entrance fee,
age 12 and under free

ELEVATION: 1,249'

RESTRICTIONS:

PETS: On leash only

FIRES: In fire rings

ALCOHOL: Prohibited in all public/
outdoor areas

VEHICLES: 2/site

OTHER: Maximum 8 people/site; guests must
leave by 10 p.m.; quiet time 10 p.m.–6 a.m.;
bring your own firewood or charcoal; limited
supplies at park store; pick up main supplies
in Boerne or San Antonio

---

of the campground, sites 16–19, 26, 29, and the 30s are also very acceptable large spaces. These sites even come with an efficient and cost-effective cleanup crew of redheaded turkey vultures, in case you forget to secure your food supplies.

Returning to the main park road, turn left and head down the hill toward the popular and usually crowded day-use area, but watch for an unassuming gravel road to your right at 0.3 mile. This turn into Wagon Ford Walk-In Tent Area offers some of the best tent camping you will find. Travel 0.2 mile to the central parking area and take your gear to any one of 9 sites, which are all secluded in a grove of huge pecan trees. The trail is level and the farthest site is less than a 10-minute walk. As a bonus, sites 90–93 are close enough for you to hear the river, but high enough on the bank for relative safety from the unpredictable Guadalupe River below. Even so, always heed the ranger's advice if Texas thunderstorms are booming in the area. There is a steep, unofficial trail to the river, but it is better to follow the nature trail toward the day-use area, enjoying the multitude of birds and Spanish moss on the trees. No matter which of these sites you get to choose, bring your rolling ice chest and stay awhile. The area includes one spigot for potable water.

Returning to the paved park road, a right turn brings you to a large parking lot and the main attraction. This heavily treed day-use area sits on the banks of one of Texas's most scenic rivers, the Guadalupe. With its cool and clear water ideal for family play, the backdrop of massive limestone cliffs blocks out the other world for a relaxing afternoon of picnicking and wading. Be sure to bring a swimsuit, sunscreen, and water shoes, along with an old-fashioned picnic lunch, to get full enjoyment of this natural wonder, but also be alert to the signs of flash flood if weather threatens.

Even on a crowded summer day, the sheer beauty of this stretch of river is sufficient to allow true relaxation. Best of all, your campsite at Wagon Ford gives you the first choice of where to spend that day.

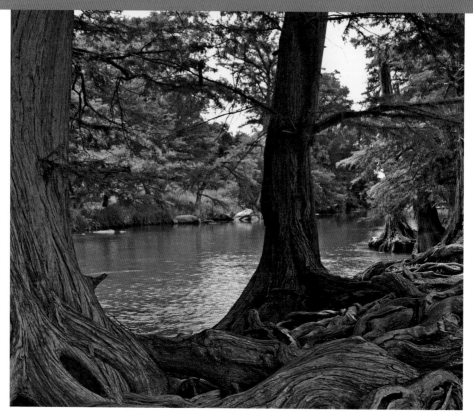
Peace and quiet in the shade

VOICES FROM THE CAMPFIRE AND RECOMMENDED READING

I come more and more to the conclusion that wilderness, in America or anywhere else, is the only thing left that is worth saving. . . . God bless America. Let's save some of it.
    Edward Abbey, *A Voice Crying in the Wilderness* (New York: St. Martin's Press, 1989).

When it was dark I set by my camp-fire smoking, and feeling pretty well satisfied; but by and by it got sort of lonesome, and so I went and set on the bank and listened to the current swashing along, and counted the stars and drift-logs and rafts that come down, and then went to bed; there ain't no better way to put in time when you are lonesome; you can't stay so, you soon get over it.
    Mark Twain, *Adventures of Huckleberry Finn* (New York, Charles L. Webster & Co., 1885).

BACKCOUNTRY ADVENTURES

While the Honey Creek tour is a great way to spend part of your day, another San Antonio–Austin area favorite is Government Canyon State Natural Area, with miles and miles of trails, including specific mountain biking areas. It also has walk-in tent-camping sites, but is only open on limited days to protect the Edwards Aquifer recharge zone and the most precious Texas resource—water. If you want to explore closer in, get a bit wet and cross to the north side of the river or take a 30-minute drive to the Bauer Unit of the park. This remote and less used area of the park isn't on the park map but includes historic structures from the late 1800s and 10 miles of nice loop hiking/equestrian trails.

BEST LOCAL FOOD AND DRINK

As the population of this historic Hill Country area continues to grow, so do the number of terrific eating establishments, ranging from upscale dining to cafés, breweries, and bistros. In Boerne, stop in Little Gretel (830-331-1368; littlegretel.com) for Czech/German dishes, O'Brien's (830-229-5600; obriensinbergheim.com) for steak and seafood, or PoPo Restaurant (830-537-4194; poporestaurant.com) for homemade American fare. In Spring Branch, try Daddy O's (830-438-0900) for great Mexican food.

Guadalupe River State Park

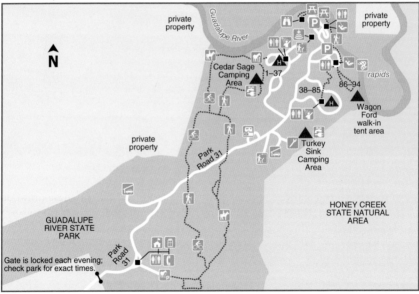

GETTING THERE

From Boerne, drive 13 miles east on TX 46. Turn left onto Park Road 31 and drive 3.2 miles to the park entrance.

GPS COORDINATES: N29° 51.198' W98° 30.264'

13

Inks Lake State Park

Beauty: ★★★ / Privacy: ★★ / Spaciousness: ★★★ / Quiet: ★★ / Security: ★★★ / Cleanliness: ★★★

The Devil's Waterhole area, with its pink, granitelike rock outcrops, is the perfect destination on a hot summer day.

Located in the heart of the Texas Hill Country, approximately 1 hour from Austin, this popular state park still manages to give the tent camper a bit of solitude and relaxation. A caveat: Avoid the RV and day-use areas on summer weekends, when the cool water acts as a magnet to every overheated Texan within driving distance. This is most evident in the Devil's Waterhole area, where the pink, granitelike rock outcrops provide natural diving platforms for the young at heart and the brave to test their nerve. While you may share this area with a small crowd, the unique beauty of this classic swimming hole makes the visit well worth the effort.

Returning to the opposite end of the park, follow the map to tent sites 300–349. This rugged and hilly area is divided into several loops, giving the sites a feeling of spaciousness and some privacy, especially on weekdays. On your immediate right, 300–304, which have level pads, make a great area for a group. Look for 304 to be nearest the water.

After another 0.3 mile on the main road, you'll reach sites 308–316. They're close to the restrooms and showers, with 311, 314, and 317 providing waterfront views and access for swimming or launching your canoe or kayak. There is nice tree cover and some brushy vegetation dividing these premium spots.

Continuing on the main road, sites 318–328 are on a rocky hillside to the left, but a right turn at 0.2 mile takes you to premium sites 332–334, which have easy water access. Also in this area, you'll find extra-large site 330, with two picnic tables. At 0.3 mile, look for the modern restrooms and showers and the park host (where you can purchase firewood) on the left, and then sites 339–343 on your right. Sites 341 and 342 are premium waterfront sites that have tree cover sufficient for hot afternoons.

Pink granite and cool water invite you to take a dip.

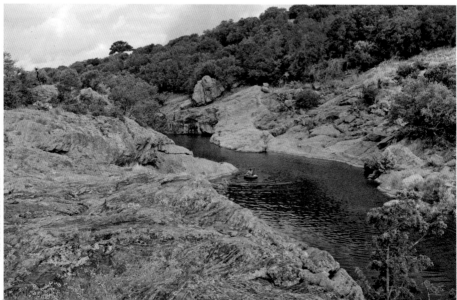

Photo credit: *Chase Fountain*

KEY INFORMATION

ADDRESS: 3630 Park Road 4, West Burnet, TX 78611

CONTACT: 512-793-2223, tpwd.texas.gov/state-parks/inks-lake

OPERATED BY: Texas Parks & Wildlife Department

OPEN: Year-round

SITES: 49 tent-only sites, Sponsored Youth Group site 3 miles from park, 50 people max (locked area, no trails or water, chemical toilet).

EACH SITE: Picnic table, fire ring, lantern hook

ASSIGNMENT: First come, first served until site-specific reservation system begins in 2018

REGISTRATION: At headquarters or reserve at texas.reserveworld.com or 512-389-8900

FACILITIES: Modern restrooms and showers, 2 fishing piers, golf course

PARKING: At each site except 244 and 246

FEE: $16/night, water only; $56 group site; $6/person entrance fee

ELEVATION: 928'

RESTRICTIONS:

PETS: On leash only. Not allowed in cabin or primitive camping area.

FIRES: In fire rings

ALCOHOL: Prohibited in all public/ outdoor areas

VEHICLES: 2/site, except 1 car only at sites 245–248

OTHER: Maximum 8 people/site; guests must leave by 10 p.m.; quiet time 10 p.m.– 6 a.m.; bring your own firewood or charcoal; limited supplies at park store; pick up main supplies in Burnet; gathering firewood prohibited

With the fishing pier on your left, the final loop contains premium lakefront sites 346– 348, which also have nice views of the lake.

As you would expect, all these lakefront sites get claimed early, so check in at headquarters first. Then you can head to the water or the well-stocked park store, or visit nearby Longhorn Cavern State Park, where its 68°F year-round temperature and guided tours are the perfect addition to your camping weekend (or week) at Inks Lake.

VOICES FROM THE CAMPFIRE AND RECOMMENDED READING

We are a great people because we have been so successful in developing and using our marvelous natural resources, but also, we Americans are the people we are largely because we have had the influence of the wilderness on our lives.

Roderick Frazier Nash *Wilderness and the American Mind* (New Haven, CT, Yale University Press, 1967).

Author's note: Congressman John P. Saylor gave this speech in 1956 to the House of Representatives.

The genius of America is greater than any candidate or any party. This campaign, hard as it has been, has not shattered my sense of humor or my sense of proportion. I still know that the fate of America cannot depend on any one man. The greatness of America is grounded in principles and not on any single personality. I, for one, shall remember that, even as President. Unless by victory we can accomplish a greater unity toward liberal effort, we shall have done little indeed.

Donald Porter Geddes, ed., *Franklin Delano Roosevelt: A Memorial* (New York, Pocket Books, 1945).

Author's note: President Franklin D. Roosevelt speaking at Madison Square Garden at the close of the 1932 campaign.

BACKCOUNTRY ADVENTURES

As with most Texas lakes, the attraction is the water, especially when summer arrives to remind us that it is really hot here. You can rent canoes and kayaks, plus swim in the many coves, but always make safety your number one priority. A headfirst dive into an unknown rocky area or forgetting your life vest can ruin more than just your holiday.

BEST LOCAL FOOD AND DRINK

After a good swim or a long hike, enjoy Bill's Burgers, Wings & Things (512-234-8216) in Burnet. If traveling south, stop at the Blue Bonnet Cafe (830-693-2344; bluebonnetcafe.net) in Marble Falls for home cooking, including breakfast all day and homemade pie. Just don't arrive too late—the pie disappears!

Inks Lake State Park

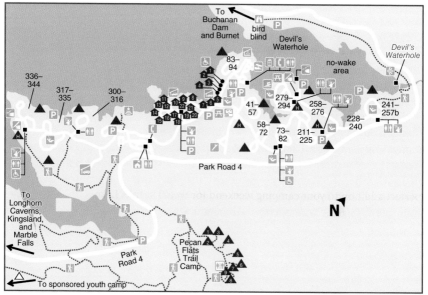

GETTING THERE

From Burnet, drive 9 miles west on TX 29. Turn left onto Park Road 4 and drive 3.4 miles before taking a right turn into the park.

GPS COORDINATES: N30° 44.202' W98° 22.200'

14

⛺ Lake Buchanan: CANYON OF THE EAGLES

Beauty: ★★★★ / Privacy: ★★★★ / Spaciousness: ★★★★ / Quiet: ★★★★ / Security: ★★★★ /
Cleanliness: ★★★★

If you want a wilderness-type experience, but need to bring along the less adventurous, Canyon of the Eagles is a perfect weekend destination.

As you leave Burnet heading west on TX 29, the Texas Hill Country views begin to unfold on the horizon. Turning right on Ranch Road 2341, this scenic winding road takes you away from civilization and dead-ends into Canyon of the Eagles. This multifunction park is part of the Lower Colorado River Authority (LCRA) system and provides a wide range of activities for the whole family.

As you enter the park on the Heart of Texas Wildlife Trail, the Eagle Eye Observatory turnoff is on your immediate right at 0.1 mile. This 0.8-mile gravel road leads to one of the darkest areas of the state and to a permanent observation area hosted by the Austin Astronomical Society. One Saturday evening each month, the observatory's retractable roof is opened to the heavens, and guests are able to peer through one of its large telescopes at such wonders as the rings of Saturn or a spectacular double star.

Returning to the main road, the entrance to Chimney Slough Campsites is across the way. These 23 sites back up to a rugged, heavily wooded area, but are nicely spaced with sites 1–3 located at the end of the road for extra privacy.

Back on the paved park road, a left turn brings you to the Bird and Butterfly Trail, which is home to the endangered golden-cheeked warbler and black-capped vireo. Continue 0.5 mile past the lodge turnoff, and the central restrooms and showers are on the left along with the RV park, where tent campers register with the park host.

Another 0.2 mile brings you to a fork in the road. To the right are the fishing pier and a group site for up to 50 campers. To the left are the Tanner Point Campground and 10

It's not the ocean, but it will do on a hot day!

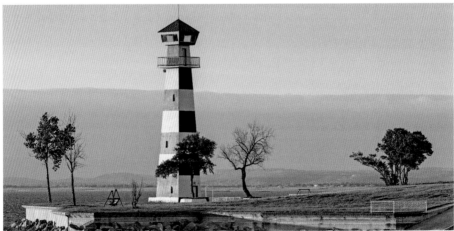

Photo credit: Shutterstock

KEY INFORMATION

ADDRESS: 16942 RR 2341,
Burnet, TX 78611

CONTACT: 512-334-2070, 800-977-0081
(reservations); canyonoftheeagles.com

OPERATED BY: LCRA/Thousand Trails

OPEN: Year-round

SITES: 33 tent, 1 group site

EACH SITE: Picnic table, fire ring

ASSIGNMENT: Reservations get you in
the campground; site choice is first come,
first served

REGISTRATION: At camp host

FACILITIES: Bring your own water for
tent sites; portable toilets nearby; modern
restrooms near lodge

PARKING: At or near each site

FEE: $25/site (Chimney Slough/park at site,
Tanner Point/walk in 100 yards); group site
$300/weekend night (Fisherman's Point
campground); $6 plus tax/person entrance
fee; $3 age 65 and older and military

ELEVATION: 1,071'

RESTRICTIONS:

PETS: On leash only

FIRES: In fire rings

ALCOHOL: Prohibited in all public/
outdoor areas

VEHICLES: 2/site

OTHER: Maximum 8 people/site; guests must
leave by 10 p.m.; quiet time 10 p.m.–6 a.m.;
bring your own firewood or charcoal; limited
supplies at park store; pick up main supplies
in Burnet

well-spaced tent sites connected by a rough gravel road. These primitive sites do not have water, but they do have a wilderness feel and sunset views that overcome any inconvenience of bringing in your own water or taking a short walk with your gear. The sounds of the birds and a cool breeze off the lake make these sites a must-stop.

For another main attraction in the area, drive two miles southeast of the park on RR 2341 and board the 70-foot Texas Eagle for the 2-hour scenic Vanishing Texas River Cruise up the Colorado River Canyon. The canyon's shores have been allowed to remain wild and offer an outdoor experience hard to duplicate in these days of waterfront developments. In the late fall and winter, these boat trips are very popular due to sightings of American bald eagles, which make this their winter home. Reservations are recommended (443 Waterway Lane, Burnet, TX 78611; 800-474-8374; vtrc.com).

As you head out of the park, don't miss the lodge area, which has great views of Lake Buchanan, a restaurant, and cozy cabins for non–tent campers. There is also live entertainment on the patio on many weekends. If you are looking for a wilderness-type experience but need to bring along the less adventurous, then Canyon of the Eagles is a perfect weekend destination.

However, if less civilization is your goal, return to TX 29, turn right, and make another right on FM 261. FM 261 follows the west shore of Lake Buchanan, and the Black Rock Park entrance is on the right at 2.7 miles. The friendly park hosts will greet you and assist with site selection, starting with sites 1–3 on your immediate right. These lakefront sites are well spaced and have excellent views of the massive Lake Buchanan. Continuing on the main park road, sites 4–11 are on your left and are slightly elevated for grand views of the lake. Site 6 is especially large with two grills and two tables. Sites 7–9 also have large shade trees for an afternoon retreat from the summer sun. Site 12 is a solo site facing east on the right near the lake, while site 13 is on the peninsula facing a sandy beach to the west. Sites 19 and 20 have huge oak trees and lake views.

While camping at Black Rock Park, keep a sharp lookout not only for great blue herons and red-tailed hawks soaring high above the lake, but also for American white pelicans and bald eagles. This area is also home to the endangered golden-cheeked warblers and black-capped vireos. Overall, this family-friendly park is a great spot to relax, throw in a fishing line, or just enjoy the serenity of Lake Buchanan just a few steps from your tent.

As you leave the park entrance, a right turn will take you to the adjacent Llano County Park and a public boat ramp. Continue north 6.9 miles to the historic Bluffton Store and make a right turn on RR 2241 for 7.3 miles. Fall Creek Vineyards (325-379-5361; fcv.com) is on your right and schedules festivals and events, such as a grape stomp, throughout the year.

Returning 3.2 miles on the main road, turn left on FM 3014 and take another left at 0.4 mile into the Cedar Point Recreation/Resource Area. This unimproved and primitive camping area has no numbered sites, but several gravel turnoffs lead to the water's edge on both sides of the peninsula. If you go to the end of the road, you arrive at a perfect waterfront site with 180-degree views of the lake and access to swimming or boating. While this site has no restrooms, showers, tables, or drinking water, it is a great getaway for tent campers looking to leave civilization behind, even for just one night.

VOICES FROM THE CAMPFIRE AND RECOMMENDED READING

In the ultimate democracy of time, Henry Thoreau has outlived his contemporaries. . . . The deeper our United States sinks into industrialism, urbanism, militarism . . . the more poignant, strong, and appealing becomes Thoreau's demand for the right of every man, every woman, every child, every dog, every tree, every snail darter, every lousewort, every living thing, to live its own life in its own way at its own pace in its own square mile of home. Or in its own stretch of river.

Edward Abbey, *Down the River with Henry Thoreau/Walden* (Layton, UT, Peregrine Smith, 1981).

The great days of America are by no means done. We have only touched the border of our achievement. If I did not believe this, I would not believe in America. Because that faith is America. So my creed, if I were asked to define it, would run something like this:

I believe in America because in it we are free—free to choose our government, to speak our minds, to observe our different religions;

Because we are generous with our freedom—we share our rights with those who disagree with us;

Because we hate no people and covet no people's lands;

Because we are blessed with a natural and varied abundance;

Because we set no limit to a man's achievement: in mine, factory, field, or service in business or the arts, an able man regardless of class or creed, can realize his ambition;

Because we have great dreams—and because we have the opportunity to make those dreams come true.

Wendell L. Willkie, "The Faith That Is America," Meet Mr. Willkie (Philadelphia, David McKay Company, 1939).

I also recommend reading *Canyon of the Eagles: A History of Lake Buchanan and Official Guide to the Vanishing Texas River Cruise* by C. L. Yarbrough (1989).

BACKCOUNTRY ADVENTURES

Lake Buchanan is a large lake that will support unlimited canoe and kayak trips. The bird-watching is plentiful, and the chance to view the American bald eagles this close to home is not to be missed. For a different type of peaceful walk, follow the new labyrinth added at the lakefront.

BEST LOCAL FOOD AND DRINK

Campers and resort guests alike are all welcome at the award-winning Overlook Restaurant in the lodge. For more simple fare, visit the recently revamped park store for good pizza or wine or a cold beer. A short drive into Burnet or another neighboring town will offer many tasty options, including barbecue, burgers, home cooking, and Mexican food.

Lake Buchanan: Canyon of the Eagles

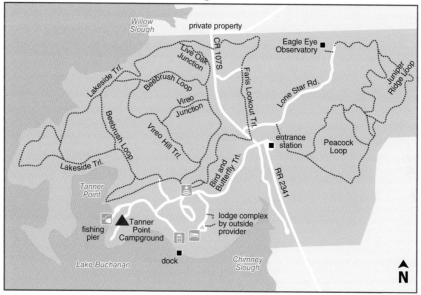

GETTING THERE

From Burnet, travel 2.7 miles west on TX 29. Turn right onto RR 2341 and drive 15.4 miles; the park is at the end of the road.

GPS COORDINATES: N30° 53.052' W98° 25.914'

15

Lake Whitney: LOFERS BEND PARK

Beauty: ★★★★ / Privacy: ★★★★ / Spaciousness: ★★★★ / Quiet: ★★★ / Security: ★★★★ / Cleanliness: ★★★

This U.S. Army Corps of Engineers property is Texas lakeside tent camping at its best.

When you leave Whitney and head west 5 miles on TX 22 toward the dam, don't miss the Lofers Park turnoff. It first appears to be a nice day-use area, but a short 0.5-mile drive and a left turn brings you to the entrance station to Lofers Bend Park (west) of Lake Whitney. The friendly gatekeepers will provide you with a map and directions to the best tent-camping sites far away from the RV area near the main boat ramp on the 49,820-acre multiuse Lake Whitney. The U.S. Army Corps of Engineers formed this lake in 1951 to provide flood control and hydroelectric power. While not generally known as a park creator, the Corps has done an excellent job in designing West Lofers with the tent camper in mind.

As you leave the entrance station, the restrooms and showers are 0.2 mile on your left; a nicely graded rock road is on your immediate right. Turn right and proceed past RV sites 1–5 and follow the ridgeline to sites 6–10. Sites 8 and 9 are toward the end of the road and provide spectacular lake views. The sites are also very well spaced and allow some real privacy. The oak tree cover provides needed shade in the summer and the lake breezes keep the air temperature pleasant even on the hottest days.

Returning to the main rock road, make a hard right toward the lake and sites 11–19. Follow the winding road and arrive at site 14 for an excellent view of the lake and a prepared tent site suitable for two tents. Sites 17–19 also have extra room and views of the lake that will have your photographers out at sunrise, sunset, and full-moon rises over the eastern horizon.

Wind power is all you need.

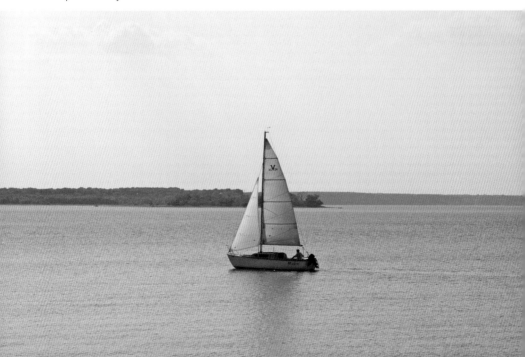

KEY INFORMATION

ADDRESS: 100 Lofers Bend Park Road, West Whitney, TX 76692

OPERATED BY: U.S. Army Corps of Engineers

CONTACT: 254-694-3189, whitney-lake.com/lofers-bend-park; reservations: 877-444-6777, recreation.gov

OPEN: Year-round

SITES: 64 in East Lofers; 67 in West Lofers; 1 group site (60 person max)

EACH SITE: Water, covered picnic table, fire ring, upright grill, lantern hook

ASSIGNMENT: Reservations available for tent sites; otherwise, first come, first served

REGISTRATION: At entrance station

FACILITIES: Modern restrooms with showers

PARKING: At each site

FEE: $12 water-only; half price with senior pass (Golden Age Passport), group site $60–$80 depending on season

ELEVATION: 557'

RESTRICTIONS:

PETS: On leash only

FIRES: In fire rings

ALCOHOL: Prohibited

VEHICLES: One RV-type vehicle/site; other vehicles not limited

OTHER: Maximum 10 people/site; guests must leave by 10 p.m.; quiet time 10 p.m.– 6 a.m.; bring your own firewood or charcoal; limited supplies at marina store; pick up main supplies in Whitney or Hillsboro

Returning on the rock road to the main park road, turn right for 0.1 mile and make an immediate right for sites 20–22. Go straight until the road ends at premium site 22, which sits at the tip of the peninsula with 180-degree views of Lake Whitney and all the people engaged in water sports passing by this elevated overlook. The site is large enough for two or three tents and offers the privacy of truly being at land's end. Remember, you can reserve sites 1–46, and site 22 will go fast any time of year.

Returning to the main road, another immediate right will get you to sites 23–27. As with the others, these sites are very well spaced for privacy and solitude. Site 26 will give you huge shade trees and a great view of the lake.

Leaving tent sites 23–27, a right turn will take you to the boat ramp and a very popular RV area. A left turn will return you to the West Lofers entrance station. Be sure to watch for bounding white-tailed deer at any time of day or night as you head straight past the marina turnoff. Of course, the marina does have a park store for emergency supplies such as cold beer. Look for the East Lofers Campground entrance ahead and receive a different map for the 64 individual sites plus 8 sites with a group camp shelter. This is primarily an RV area, but sites 33–38 are nonelectric sites at lake level that allow you to pull your boat up to the shoreline. There's not much shade, but site 36 puts you out on the waterfront with the sound of waves and wind at your tent's front porch.

Be sure to check with the entrance station before heading toward the water-level campsites. While the Texas drought makes these sites high and dry, flooding can result in these lower sites being under multiple feet of water.

VOICES FROM THE CAMPFIRE AND RECOMMENDED READING

Yet, at the very moment that the bond is breaking between the young and the natural world, a growing body of research links our mental, physical, and spiritual health directly to our

association with nature—in positive ways. Several of these studies suggest that thoughtful exposure of youngsters to nature can even be a powerful form of therapy for attention-deficit disorders and other maladies. As one scientist puts it, we can now assume that just as children need good nutrition and adequate sleep, they may very well need contact with nature.

Richard Louv, *Last Child in the Woods* (Chapel Hill, NC, Algonquin Books of Chapel Hill, 2008).

BACKCOUNTRY ADVENTURES

While the motorboat and Sea-Doo crowds are out in full force on summer weekends, this huge lake allows canoes, kayaks, and sailboats to have more than enough space for a day of exploration and enjoyment.

BEST LOCAL FOOD AND DRINK

In addition to the well-loved Texas Great Country Cafe & Pie Pantry (254-694-3608; texasgreatcountrycafe.com), the Hooten Holler'n BBQ (254-694-4030) in Whitney will fill you up after a busy day outdoors. If you don't mind the outlet mall traffic in Hillsboro, locals enjoy home-style cooking at Lone Star Cafe (254-582-2030), Taylor's Smokehouse (254-266-4209), and A Tiskit A Taskit (254-582-3807), a classic soda joint.

Lake Whitney: Lofers Bend Park

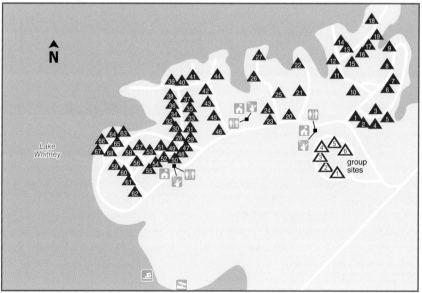

GETTING THERE

From Hillsboro and Interstate 35, travel 18 miles west on TX 22. The park is on the right, just before the dam.

GPS COORDINATES: N31° 52.782' W97° 21.816'

16

Lake Whitney State Park

Beauty: ★★★★ / Privacy: ★★★ / Spaciousness: ★★★ / Quiet: ★★★ / Security: ★★★★ / Cleanliness: ★★★

A great photo op for sunsets, great blue herons, and even redheaded turkey vultures soaring above.

The surrounding rolling ranchland does not really prepare you for this lake, with 23,550 surface acres and 70 tent sites to choose from. As you pass the entrance station on the Prairies and Pineywoods Wildlife Trail West, proceed straight for 0.4 mile until you turn right at the Horseshoe Loop. The tent sites begin at 18, with covered picnic tables on the even-numbered side, which backs up to a heavily wooded area. Continue on the loop road until you see sites 39–46, which have nice tree cover and a little extra distance from the RV area.

Return to the main road and proceed 0.5 mile until you see the hiking trailhead on your right. This round-trip walk in the park of 0.9 mile will give you a nice bit of exercise, but do pay attention to the warning signs advising that snakes may be waiting on the trail to welcome you. Of course, when it's 106°F on a late-July afternoon, the snakes are probably at the lake, which is where you should head next. Proceeding on the main road, the boat ramp is on your immediate right and the swimming area is only 0.3 mile farther. Please note the emphasis on water safety, given the rash of drownings at Texas lakes.

Returning to the main road and the beginning of Park Road 47, White-Tail sites 52–68 have lake views with covered picnic tables, running water, and some nice trees. Look for site 59, which is not only close to the water but also large enough for your family and sheltered by a massive shade tree.

Who needs trees when you have lakefront camping?

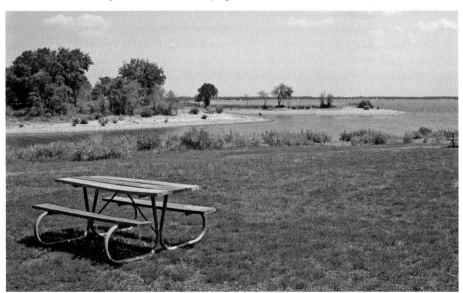

KEY INFORMATION

ADDRESS: FM 1244, Whitney, TX 76692

CONTACT: 254-694-3793,
tpwd.texas.gov/state-parks/lake-whitney

OPERATED BY: Texas Parks & Wildlife
Department

OPEN: Year-round

SITES: 63 tent sites; Sponsored Youth Group
site (24 person max, no water)

EACH SITE: Picnic table, central water,
fire ring

ASSIGNMENT: First come, first served
until site-specific reservation system
begins in 2018

REGISTRATION: At headquarters or reserve
at texas.reserveworld.com or
512-389-8900

FACILITIES: Centrally located showers and
modern restrooms

PARKING: At each site

FEE: $14 water-only sites; $5/person entrance
fee ages 13–65; $2/person age 65 and
older; youth group site $30 when available

ELEVATION: 836'

RESTRICTIONS:

PETS: On leash only

FIRES: In fire rings

ALCOHOL: Prohibited in all public/
outdoor areas

VEHICLES: 2/site

OTHER: Some areas/facilities previously
closed while repairs made due to flood
damage—contact park for updates; maximum 8 people/site; guests must leave by
10 p.m.; quiet time 10 p.m.–6 a.m.; limited
supplies at park store, including firewood;
pick up main supplies in Whitney or Hillsboro; gathering firewood prohibited

Turning right for 0.2 mile, you'll come upon Star View sites 69–86, which lead you back toward the lake, with sites 76–79 nearest the waterfront. Back on the park road, proceed 0.3 mile, where you'll find the new restrooms and showers on your left. At 0.5 mile, the primitive group campground is on the right. Your eager young campers won't find any shade, but the lake view is super.

The final tent campgrounds are Lakeview/Sunset Ridge sites 111–137. The lakefront sites (111–123) are made even more attractive by a short rock road directly to the lake's edge and a great photography spot for sunsets, great blue herons, and even a redheaded turkey vulture soaring above. Be sure to continue through Sunset Ridge and take the road that ends at the lake. This wide-open area has a coastal feel, and a private walk on the beach will be a great way to end your tent-camping visit.

As you leave the park, watch for the 2,000-foot airstrip near the deer-crossing sign. If you happen to own a private plane, you can keep your camping gear packed for a quick return to your favorite site and more Lake Whitney beauty.

VOICES FROM THE CAMPFIRE AND RECOMMENDED READING

Conservation is a state of harmony between men and land. . . . It is inconceivable to me that an ethical relation to land can exist without love, respect, and admiration for land, and a high regard for its value. By value, I of course mean something far broader than mere economic value; I mean value in the philosophical sense.

Aldo Leopold, *A Sand County Almanac* (Oxford, United Kingdom, Oxford University Press, 1949).

The shift in our relationship to the natural word is startling, even in settings that one would assume are devoted to nature. Not that long ago, summer camp was a place where you camped, hiked in the woods, learned about plants and animals, or told firelight stories about ghosts or mountain lions. As likely as not today, "summer camp" is a weight-loss camp, or a computer camp. For a new generation, nature is more abstraction than reality. Increasingly, nature is something to watch, to consume, to wear—to ignore.

Richard Louv, *Last Child in the Woods* (Chapel Hill, NC, Algonquin Books of Chapel Hill, 2008).

BACKCOUNTRY ADVENTURES

The lakeside tent sites here are a nice treat when you are still a few hundred miles from the Texas coast. The west-facing sites are great for sunset cookouts and usually have a strong breeze to lower the temperature inside your tent. The lake is plenty big for all forms of boating, so be prepared for a little motor noise on summer weekends. Otherwise, a canoe, kayak, or small fishing boat will let you find a quiet cove for just you and the birds.

BEST LOCAL FOOD AND DRINK

Texas Great Country Cafe & Pie Pantry (254-694-3608; texasgreatcountrycafe.com) is a not-to-be-missed treat, offering breakfast all day, a full menu, amazing pie, and a great cup of coffee. Montes Breakfast Burritos (254-694-3279) is also a local favorite in Whitney.

Lake Whitney State Park

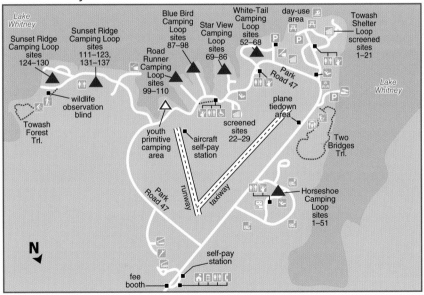

GETTING THERE

From I-35 in Hillsboro, travel 13 miles west on TX 22. Turn right onto FM 1244. The park is 2.4 miles ahead.

GPS COORDINATES: N31° 55.866' W97° 21.414'

17

McKinney Falls State Park

Beauty: ★★★★ / Privacy: ★★★ / Spaciousness: ★★★ / Quiet: ★★★ / Security: ★★★★ / Cleanliness: ★★★★

Watch for mule deer out for a late-afternoon snack and return often to this urban oasis.

Located less than 45 minutes from the bright lights and eclectic music scene of downtown Austin, this hidden retreat will soothe those big-city nerves in a hurry. Located just 2 miles west of US 183 on McKinney Falls Parkway, the park will take you back in time to when Central Texas was the home of American Indians and the early pioneers were looking for a patch of farmland and dependable water.

After leaving the headquarters, an immediate right turn leads 0.4 mile to Lower McKinney Falls parking area and trailhead. From here, an easy five-minute walk takes you to one of the area's most popular warm-weather destinations. The open expanses of smooth limestone and emerald-green pools invite swimming, wading, or just enjoying the small waterfall. Of course, this area can quickly change its character if thunderstorms are booming on the horizon. This area also marks the beginning of the 2.8-mile Homestead Trail for hikers and mountain bikers. As you leave the Lower Falls area, also note the parking on your right for the Picnic Trail day-use area for a little privacy off the paved road.

Returning to the main road, another right turn for 0.3 mile leads to the Upper McKinney Falls and the Smith Visitor Center and Viewpoint. This scenic part of the park is very

McKinney Falls is beautiful, even at low water.

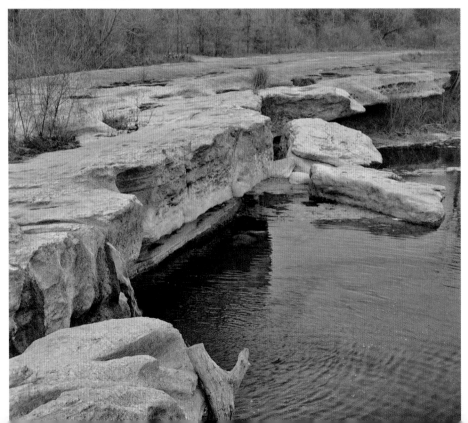

KEY INFORMATION

ADDRESS: 5808 McKinney Falls Pkwy., Austin, TX 78744

CONTACT: 512-243-1643, tpwd.texas.gov/state-parks/mckinney-falls

OPERATED BY: Texas Parks & Wildlife Department

OPEN: Year-round

SITES: 8 tent-only; 81 with water and electricity; Sponsored Youth Primitive Group area, 50 person max, water and restrooms nearby

EACH SITE: Picnic table, fire ring, lantern ring

ASSIGNMENT: First come, first served until site-specific reservation system begins in 2018

REGISTRATION: At headquarters or reserve at texas.reserveworld.com or 512-389-8900

FACILITIES: Modern restrooms with showers

PARKING: Central parking; 5- to 10-minute walk to tent sites

FEE: $20–$24 for tent sites; $6/person entrance fee; $75 Youth Primitive Group area

ELEVATION: 552'

RESTRICTIONS:

PETS: On leash only

FIRES: In fire rings, but check for burn bans

ALCOHOL: Prohibited in all public/outdoor areas

VEHICLES: 2/site

OTHER: Maximum 4 people and one tent/site; guests must leave by 10 p.m.; quiet time 10 p.m.–6 a.m.; bring your own firewood or charcoal; limited supplies at park store; pick up main supplies in Austin; gathering firewood prohibited

---

popular, with access to the 1-mile Rock Shelter Interpretive Trail and the 2.8-mile Onion Creek Hike and Bike Trail, which circles the various campgrounds.

Following the main road to the right from the visitor center for 0.4 mile, turn right into the walk-in primitive camping area and the modern restrooms. This unassuming entrance quickly leads down a short incline to the Onion Creek Hike and Bike Trail, with towering shade trees along the creek bank. To the right are picnic areas. To the left are eight premium waterfront tent sites with a sense of relaxation far removed from the nearby big city. Look for sites 2, 4, 5, and 8 for the most-level tent pads. Also, bring your bike or walking shoes, since the Onion Creek Trail is just a few steps away.

Back on the main road for 0.2 mile, the Shelter Area and Youth Group Area are on your right and the Grapevine Loop Camping (trailer/RV area) is another 0.1 mile. While this area is not ideal for tent camping, look for sites 41–84, as many of these have large, level tent pads next to the parking spots and would certainly be better than missing out on this fine state park.

VOICES FROM THE CAMPFIRE AND RECOMMENDED READING

Let me say a word or two in favor of the habit of keeping a journal of one's thoughts and days.... It is a sort of deposit account wherein one saves up bits and fragments of his life that would otherwise be lost to him.

Ann Ronald, ed., "John Burroughs," Words for the Wild: The Sierra Club Trailside Reader (San Francisco, Sierra Club, 1987).

The man who publishes a book is a man with a sending set but no receiver, broadcasting messages into space without ever knowing whether they have reached any ears. He writes his

name and corks it into a bottle that he sets afloat on the ocean in the hope that some pen pal, somewhere, on whatever unpredictable coast, will find it. He drops his feather into the Grand Canyon and stands expectantly, waiting for the crash.
Wallace Stegner, *On Teaching and Writing Fiction* (New York, Penguin Books, 2002).

BACKCOUNTRY ADVENTURES

The Homestead Trail and the Onion Creek Hike & Bike Trail offer some wide-open space to get a little exercise, then enjoy a cool dip below the falls. While it's hard to get a wilderness experience near the big city, taking a trip here on a weekday afternoon is better than sitting in a car on the interstate wondering what happened to the Austin of our memories.

BEST LOCAL FOOD AND DRINK

Nearby Austin offers an abundance of eateries, as eclectic and varied as those fortunate to live in this area of Texas. A few highly rated options closer to the park include the Bouldin Creek Cafe (512-416-1601; bouldincreekcafe.com) for delicious vegetarian breakfasts, Home Slice Pizza (512-444-7437; homeslicepizza.com), and Matt's El Rancho (512-462-9333; mattselrancho.com) or Tacodeli (512-732-0303; tacodeli.com) for Mexican dishes.

McKinney Falls State Park

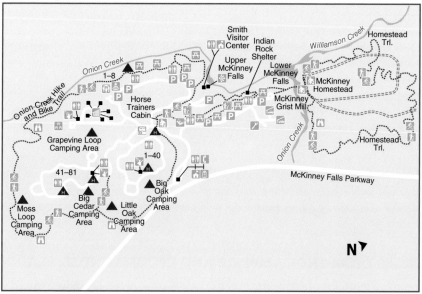

GETTING THERE

From Austin, take East Seventh Street and US 183 southeast about 7 miles to McKinney Falls Parkway. Turn right and drive 2.7 miles to the park entrance on the right.

GPS COORDINATES: N30° 10.836' W97° 43.332'

18

Meridian State Park

Beauty: ★★★★ / Privacy: ★★★★ / Spaciousness: ★★★★ / Quiet: ★★★★ / Security: ★★★★ / Cleanliness: ★★★

Don't miss the brilliant lake views in this sought-after destination.

As you enter the town of Meridian, the peaceful pace of a small town immediately draws you in. The 1886 courthouse sits on the square surrounded by small shops, little changed for more than a century. A faded road sign announces you are at the "Top of the Hill Country" and in the home of the "World's Best Barbecue Cook-Off." For Texans, this is a good omen.

Leaving town on TX 22, head west and cross the Bosque River. The entrance to Meridian State Park is 2.6 miles on the right. After you turn into the entrance, park headquarters is 0.1 mile ahead. Continue straight ahead for sites 16–23 on the right. These sites are sheltered by heavy tree cover and back up to a rocky streambed that could fill up quickly in a typical Texas cloudburst. The sites have good spacing but get a little road noise from the state highway.

As you continue on the main park road, a low-water crossing and a scenic, hilly, winding road is a reminder of why the Hill Country is such a sought-after destination. The tree cover and thick vegetation come to the edge of the road, with tight turns giving you a glimpse of the lake far below on your right. As you begin your downhill route, watch for a small rock bridge and site 24 shaded by huge cottonwood trees. This solo site is large enough for multiple tents and sits at the edge of a small inlet for the lake. The lake view is excellent and there are no other tents or RVs in sight. You won't have water, electricity, or modern restrooms, but this site is so special that these small inconveniences are no problem.

Leaving site 24, continue for 0.2 mile and watch for an unmarked, paved turnoff on your right. A moderately steep approach will bring you down to a gravel parking lot and lakefront

CCC stonework at its best

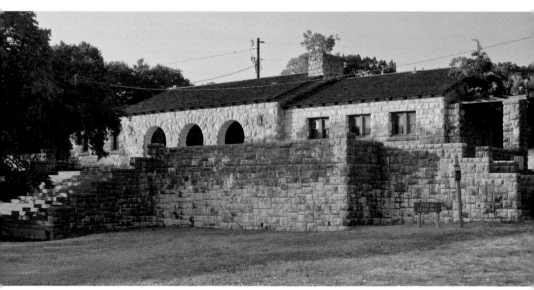

KEY INFORMATION

ADDRESS: 173 Park Road 7,
Meridian, TX 76665

CONTACT: 254-435-2536,
tpwd.texas.gov/state-parks/meridian

OPERATED BY: Texas Parks & Wildlife
Department

OPEN: Year-round

SITES: 16 tent-only sites,
1 group primitive area (site 32)

EACH SITE: 16–23 have water only;
24–31 have no water

ASSIGNMENT: First come, first served
until site-specific reservation system
begins in 2018

REGISTRATION: At headquarters or reserve
at texas.reserveworld.com or
512-389-8900

FACILITIES: Restrooms and showers near
shelters and lake

PARKING: At each site

FEE: $15–$17; $5/person entrance fee;
age 12 and under free

ELEVATION: 977'

RESTRICTIONS:

PETS: On leash only

FIRES: Check with headquarters for burn ban

ALCOHOL: Prohibited in all public/
outdoor areas

VEHICLES: 2/site

OTHER: Maximum 8 people/site; guests must
leave by 10 p.m.; quiet time 10 p.m.–
6 a.m.; limited supplies at headquarters;
pick up main supplies in Meridian;
gathering firewood prohibited

sites 30 and 31. These premier spots have an unobstructed view of the lake, large trees, and privacy enough for your entire family or group. The sun sets behind you and you can watch the brilliant colors reflected over the water to the far shoreline. The breeze blows even on the hottest summer evenings, and the birds welcome you to their hidden part of the park.

Returning to the main road, turn right for 0.5 mile of steady elevation gain until you reach the Shinnery Ridge trailhead. This 1.64-mile trail is mostly rough and unspoiled, but the last portion is paved for easy walking and wheelchair access. As you enjoy this area, watch for the usual suspects such as skunks and raccoons, but also try to spot ringtail cats and opossums.

Returning on the park road for 1.3 miles, the main park area contains the historic rock structures, picnic areas, and shelters near the swimming cove. Continue 0.2 mile on the one-way road until you reach group site 32. This grassy area is also lakefront property and shaded by huge trees and holds up to 8 tents.

As you continue on the park road, the lake is on your left and sheer rock walls are on the right. The Bee Ledge Scenic Lookout is 0.7 mile on your left and is an excellent photography viewpoint for sunsets. As you return to the entrance, watch for roadrunners and white-tailed deer sprinting across the road.

VOICES FROM THE CAMPFIRE AND RECOMMENDED READING

This is a delicious evening, when the whole body is one sense, and imbibes delight through every pore. I go and come with a strange liberty in Nature.
Henry David Thoreau, *Walden, or Life in the Woods* (Boston, Ticknor and Fields, 1854).

BACKCOUNTRY ADVENTURES

The Meridian hiking trails and quiet lake are nice ways to get off the road, but the real adventure here is in the solitude and paying attention to details. Below the earthen dam is a geology field trip cut through by a biology water lab. This area can be reached through the campsite number 16–18. A second place to stop and contemplate is the park road to Bee Ledge Lookout. While you can drive this uphill route, I suggest an easy trek up from near campsite 32 to the lookout. Along the way, the geology contains massive limestone overhangs with a nice family of turkey vultures relaxing in the cool shadows waiting for dinnertime. A lesson we can all learn.

BEST LOCAL FOOD AND DRINK

For everything from burgers, to Mexican food, to chicken fried steak, to bread pudding, make a stop at the Cactus Grill (254-435-6062), which serves homemade selections a local describes as "country fine dining." If you're driving via I-35 through the town of West, enjoy a meal at Slovacek's (254-826-4525; slovacekwesttexas.com) or the Czech-American Restaurant (254-826-3008), or pick up kolache and other bakery items from the Czech Stop (254-826-5316; czechstop.net).

Meridian State Park

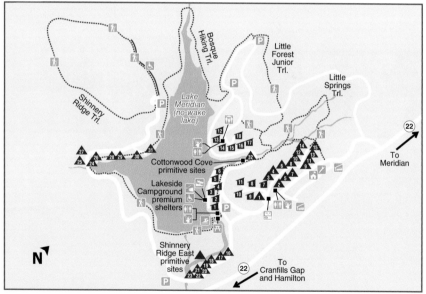

GETTING THERE

From Meridian, go west on TX 22 for 4 miles. The park is on the right.

GPS COORDINATES: N31° 53.454' W97° 41.850'

19

⛺ Palmetto State Park

Beauty: ★★★ / Privacy: ★★★ / Spaciousness: ★★★★ / Quiet: ★★★★ / Security: ★★★ / Cleanliness: ★★

Premium sites here sit on a peninsula formed by a bend in the wild and scenic San Marcos River.

Surrounded by early Texas history, Palmetto State Park is 10 miles north of Gonzales, where one of the most famous events on the road to the Alamo occurred, which led to the eventual independence of Texas. On October 2, 1835, just 5 miles southwest of Gonzales on TX 97, the first shot in the Texas Revolution was fired after a group of 18 Texans refused to comply with 150 Mexican dragoons who demanded they turn over their only cannon. The Texans' response of "come and take it" has been a part of military history and Texas legend ever since.

After traveling 10.6 miles north from Gonzales on US 183 through rugged ranch land, a left turn onto Park Road 11 leads to a scenic overlook of the entire valley for perfect sunset pictures. The trees start to close in over the descending road as you approach the village of Ottine. Park headquarters is on your right, and the Warm Springs Hospital Complex looms on the left with a distinct feeling of the 1930s and 1940s.

After leaving the headquarters, continue 0.2 mile and turn left along Oxbow Lake into the camping area. Shaded by large oaks covered with Spanish moss, sites 20–24 back up to

This water tower was built by the CCC.

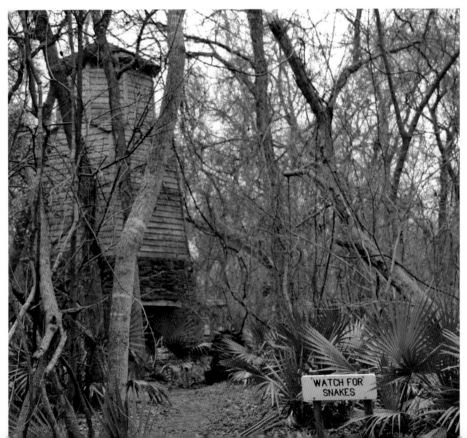

KEY INFORMATION

ADDRESS: 78 Park Road 11 S, Gonzales, TX 78629

CONTACT: 830-672-3266, tpwd.texas.gov/state-parks/palmetto

OPERATED BY: Texas Parks & Wildlife Department

OPEN: Year-round

SITES: 20

EACH SITE: Picnic table, upright grill, fire ring, lantern hook

ASSIGNMENT: First come, first served until site-specific reservation system begins in 2018

REGISTRATION: At headquarters or self-registration station or reserve at texas.reserveworld.com or 512-389-8900

FACILITIES: Modern restrooms with showers in RV area, park store

PARKING: At each site

FEE: $12 water-only sites; $3/person entrance fee; 12 and under free. Group camping area (100 people/25 car max, $60, water at site, restrooms nearby)

ELEVATION: 302'

RESTRICTIONS:

PETS: On leash only

FIRES: In fire rings

ALCOHOL: Prohibited in all public/outdoor areas

VEHICLES: 2/site

OTHER: Maximum 8 people/site; guests must leave by 10 p.m.; quiet time 10 p.m.–6 a.m.; bring your own firewood or charcoal; limited supplies at park store; pick up main supplies in Gonzales or Luling; gathering firewood prohibited

a small lake with a playground to the left. Continuing on, sites 38–40 surround an artesian well and pond where the local ducks provide the entertainment, along with canoes and paddleboats in season.

Returning to the main road, a right turn takes you deeper into the woods and onto a wide peninsula formed by a bend in the wild and scenic San Marcos River. Sites 25–33 are well spaced and back up to heavy brush until you reach the premium sites 34–40, which offer river views from a bluff and also enough room to spread out.

After these sites, there is a low-water crossing to the group camping area straight ahead, and also a paved trail to the left that crosses the river to the group pavilion known as the CCC Refectory. This area is also accessible by car if you return to Park Road 11, turn left and go 0.5 mile, cross three small bridges, and turn left again.

As you approach the refectory, you pass through backwater areas of palmetto plants, which seem out of place in this part of Texas, but still thrive in this environment of heat, humidity, and heavy spring rainfall. After you park, return to the Palmetto Trail, but do watch for snakes and poison ivy, which also enjoy this tropical paradise. Be sure to pick up the Palmetto and River Nature trails guidebook at the trailhead. This small pamphlet will enhance your visit and give an excellent description of the wide variety of trees and understory plants here, including Carolina wolfberry, Alabama supplejack, trumpet creeper, and of course, dwarf palmetto. It is worthwhile to make a special stop to see the hydraulic ram pump, which was installed in 1936 to provide Civilian Conservation Corps (CCC) workers and park visitors with drinking water. This nonelectric marvel was powered by the artesian well below it and reminds us of the valuable remote work performed by these hardy workers during the Great Depression.

Upon leaving the trail, return to the parking lot to visit one of Texas's finest CCC buildings. Known as the refectory or the Concession Building, its original roof was covered with thousands of palmetto leaves and served as the center of CCC camp activity, which included the luxurious provision of regular food, medical, and dental care for the workers. Of particular note, many CCC "boys" actually gained weight, despite their backbreaking labor. As you view this impressive stone structure and its perch overlooking the river, you will come to fully appreciate the CCC workers' contributions to Texas State Parks and FDR's vision of the CCC.

VOICES FROM THE CAMPFIRE AND RECOMMENDED READING

The Alamo was one of the earliest of these establishments . . . a mere wreck of its former grandeur. . . . The church-door opens on the square, and is meagerly decorated by stucco mouldings, all hacked and battered in the battles it has seen. Since the heroic defense of Travis and his handful of men in '36, it has been a monument, not so much to faith as to courage.
   Frederick Law Olmsted, *A Journey Through Texas* (New York, Dix, Edwards & Co., 1857).

The idea of wilderness needs no defense. It only needs more defenders.
   Edward Abbey, *The Journey Home: Some Words in Defense of the American West* (New York, Dutton, 1977).

BACKCOUNTRY ADVENTURES

Canoe trips are a popular way to see the San Marcos River as it flows toward Gonzales. These leisurely trips also give you time to contemplate the historic legacy of being a Texan,

The refectory is one of the finest examples of CCC work in Texas.

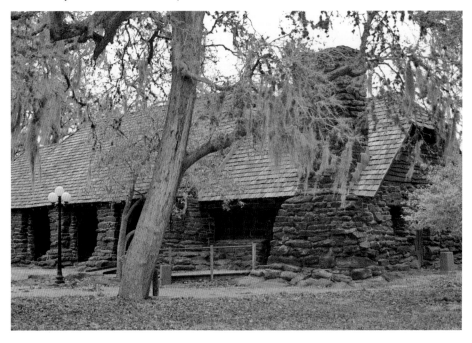

either native or newly arrived. From that first shot at Gonzales, the massacre at Goliad, the Battle of the Alamo, and the final Battle of San Jacinto, Texans of both Mexican and European descent have been born with historical bloodlines of courage. With that courage, Texans must now fight even harder to protect the land that created us all.

BEST LOCAL FOOD AND DRINK

While in Luling, order sausage or other picks from a full menu at City Market (830-875-9019; lulingcitymarket.com) and indulge your guilty side with homemade onion rings worth the drive. Or get mouthwatering barbecue at Blake's Cafe (830-875-6086) or Luling Bar-B-Q (830-875-3848; lulingbar-b-q.com).

Palmetto State Park

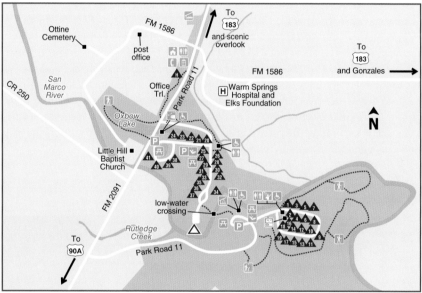

GETTING THERE

From Gonzales, travel 10.6 miles north on US 183. Turn left onto PR 11 and drive about 2 miles. Park headquarters will be on the right.

From Luling, travel 6 miles south on US 183. Turn right onto PR 11 and drive about 2 miles. Park headquarters will be on the right.

GPS COORDINATES: N29° 35.784' W97° 35.082'

20

⚠ Pedernales Falls State Park

Beauty: ★★★★ / Privacy: ★★★ / Spaciousness: ★★★ / Quiet: ★★★ / Security: ★★★★ / Cleanliness: ★★★

Don't miss the scenic overlook of massive rocks smoothed by the river's incredible force in this Hill Country escape.

As you head west from Austin on US 290, you quickly leave the traffic and bright lights of the state's capital and begin a journey into Texas history. The 38-mile scenic drive brings you to Pedernales Falls State Park, and a sense of remoteness will have you rolling down your car windows and soaking up the smells of the Texas Hill Country.

After leaving the entrance station, an immediate elevation drop brings you closer to the Pedernales River. A right turn at 0.3 mile leads to the parking area for the primitive camping area, an easy 2-mile backpack on Wolf Mountain Trail, which also allows mountain bikers. Continue on the main road 0.5 mile, and turn right for the main camping area. It has well-spaced campsites that allow both RVs and tents, but the two groups seem to voluntarily separate themselves. The tent campers tend to gather near the nature trail and sites 14–31. The sites on the right back up to the river bluff, which is high enough for safety but close enough to access the river on Trammels Crossing, a short 10-minute walk to the river's edge. The trailhead is next to sites 32 and 34 and descends to the cool, clear waters for wading or shallow swimming. Be sure to bring your water shoes and any other picnic supplies so you can spend the afternoon relaxing on this legendary river.

This is a great viewpoint unless the flood warnings are up.

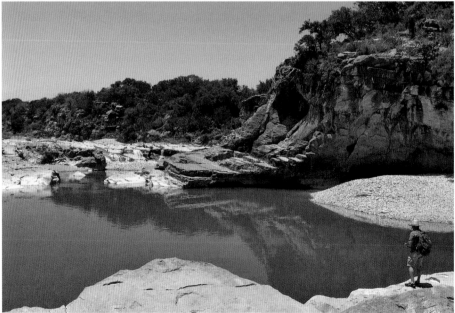

Photo credit: *Shutterstock*

KEY INFORMATION

ADDRESS: 2585 Park Road 6026, Johnson City, TX 78636

OPERATED BY: Texas Parks & Wildlife Department

CONTACT: 800-792-1112 or 830-868-7304, tpwd.texas.gov/state-parks/pedernales-falls

OPEN: Year-round

SITES: 66; one sponsored youth group area (150 people max)

EACH SITE: Picnic tables, water, fire ring, lantern hook, electricity; youth group site has picnic tables and a chemical toilet nearby

ASSIGNMENT: First come, first served until site-specific reservation system begins in 2018

REGISTRATION: At headquarters/entrance station or reserve at texas.reserveworld.com or 512-389-8900

FACILITIES: Modern restrooms and shower

PARKING: At each site

FEE: $20; $6/person entrance fee; youth group site $75

ELEVATION: 1,029'

RESTRICTIONS:

PETS: on leash only

FIRES: In fire rings only; check for burn bans

ALCOHOL: Prohibited in all public/outdoor areas

VEHICLES: 2/site

OTHER: Maximum 8 people/site; guests must leave by 10 p.m.; quiet time 10 p.m.–6 a.m.; bring your own firewood or charcoal; limited supplies at park store; pick up main supplies in Austin or Johnson City; gathering firewood prohibited

After you make camp, return to the main road and turn right for 1.4 miles toward Pedernales Falls. From the main parking lot, a leisurely 15-minute walk will bring you to a scenic overlook of the massive rocks smoothed by the river's incredible force during rainy periods. Be sure to read the flash flood warning sign and follow ranger instructions if you plan to walk out into the riverbed. Due to water danger along this unpredictable section of the river, swimming or wading is prohibited.

Upon leaving the park, head west on Ranch Road 2766 for 9.3 miles to Johnson City and begin your tour of the Lyndon B. Johnson National Historical Park at LBJ's boyhood home. Travel 14 miles farther west on US 290 and visit the LBJ Ranch, which has been restored to look much as it did when LBJ was the 36th president. Along with his wife, Lady Bird, he entertained national and world leaders on the rocky banks of the Pedernales River.

As you enjoy this tranquil riverside setting, it's easy to see why LBJ used his ranch as a retreat from the stress of politics. It's also easy to imagine the raging Pedernales River and the parallels to LBJ's inner battles to solve the nation's seemingly unsolvable problems. Whatever the mood of the river on your visit, this Hill Country escape is a required stop.

VOICES FROM THE CAMPFIRE AND RECOMMENDED READING

I wasn't looking for grizzlies but found them anyway. What was invaluable was the way the bears dominated the psychic landscape. After Vietnam, nothing less would anchor the attention. The grizzly instilled enforced humility; you were living with a creature of great beauty married to mystery who could chew your ass off anytime it chose.

Doug Peacock, *Walking it Off: A Veteran's Chronicle of War and Wilderness* (Spokane, Eastern Washington University Press, 2005).

If people persist in trespassing upon the grizzlies' territory, we must accept the fact that the grizzlies, from time to time, will harvest a few trespassers.
Edward Abbey, *A Voice Crying in the Wilderness* (New York: St. Martin's Press, 1989).

BACKCOUNTRY ADVENTURES

The best way to get away in this popular park is to take the Wolf Mountain Trail on foot or by mountain bike. The overnight site is a good place for beginning backpackers. Return by way of the river, where swimming and floating are still allowed downstream from the falls.

BEST LOCAL FOOD AND DRINK

While visiting Johnson City, relax with flavorful food at East Main Grill (830-868-7710) or Bryans on 290 (830-868-2424; bryanson290.com), or food, craft beer, and sometimes live music at Pecan Street Brewing (830-868-2500; pecanstreetbrewing.com). Rolling in Thyme & Dough (512-894-0001; thymeanddough.com), Crepe Crazy Cafe (512-524-3198; crepecrazy .com), and Creek Road Café (512-858-9459; creekroadcafe.com) are a few of the sites for tasty offerings in Dripping Springs.

Pedernales Falls State Park

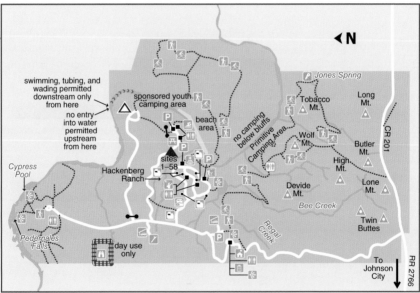

GETTING THERE

From Austin, drive 32 miles west on US 290. Turn right onto Ranch Road 3232 and drive 6.4 miles. Turn right onto Pedernales Falls Road, and almost immediately the park entrance will be on your right.

From Johnson City, drive 9.3 miles east on RR 2766.

GPS COORDINATES: N30° 18.468' W98° 15.450'

NORTH CENTRAL TEXAS AND THE LAKE COUNTRY

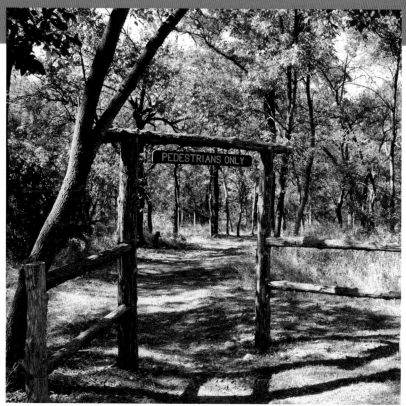

A tree-shaded hike can't be beat. (Eisenhower State Park: Lake Texoma; see page 86)

21

Dinosaur Valley State Park

Beauty: ★★★ / Privacy: ★★ / Spaciousness: ★★★★ / Quiet: ★★★ / Security: ★★★★ / Cleanliness: ★★★★

A perfect place to introduce the entire family to tent camping.

Located less than 2 hours from the crowded freeways, glass towers, and suburban sprawl of Dallas–Fort Worth, this weekend getaway is a perfect place to introduce the entire family to tent camping. The park contains 1,523 acres of wide-ranging vegetation (oaks and Ashe junipers in the upland areas and cedar elms in the creek bottoms) across a varied terrain, creating excellent opportunities for day hikes, mountain bike trails, and equestrian areas, and features the real attraction and the park's namesake, a home for dinosaurs. Well, at least dinosaur tracks. These rare and clearly preserved tracks are located mainly at four areas, which are easily accessible depending on the water flow of the clear and cool Paluxy River. The river runs through the park, exposing the tracks in its riverbed. The importance of these sites was recognized by the National Park Service, which designated it as a National Natural Landmark.

First discovered in 1909, the tracks received little attention until 1938, when Roland T. Bird of the American Museum of Natural History visited the site and identified a remarkable double set of tracks left by a giant brontosaurus-like sauropod being followed, maybe pursued, by a large carnivorous dinosaur. While these incredible prints were excavated and hauled off to New York, the park still contains excellent tracks of giant three-toed birds,

An easy crossing at low water leads to great hiking; photo credit: *Shutterstock*

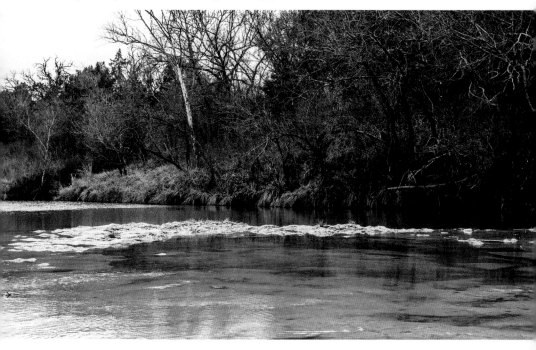

KEY INFORMATION

ADDRESS: 1629 Park Road 59, Glen Rose, TX 76043

CONTACT: 254-897-4588, tpwd.texas.gov/state-parks/dinosaur-valley

OPERATED BY: Texas Parks & Wildlife Department

OPEN: Year-round

SITES: 46

EACH SITE: Picnic table, fireplace, electric hookup, hanging pole, water tap

ASSIGNMENT: First come, first served until site-specific reservation system begins in 2018

REGISTRATION: At entrance station or reserve at texas.reserveworld.com or 512-389-8900

FACILITIES: Central bathroom with showers

PARKING: At sites and trailhead for North Primitive Camping Area

FEE: $25; $7/person entrance fee, age 12 and under free

ELEVATION: 778'

RESTRICTIONS:

PETS: On leash only

FIRES: In fireplaces/grates only

ALCOHOL: Prohibited in all public/ outdoor areas

VEHICLES: No limits

OTHER: Maximum 8 people/site; guests must leave by 10 p.m.; quiet time 10 p.m.– 6 a.m.; bring your own firewood or charcoal; limited snacks and drinks at gift shop; pick up other supplies in Glen Rose

two-legged carnosaurs, early ancestors of the Tyrannosaurus rex, and the sauropods, which were 30–50 feet long and apparently a tasty meal for the local T. rex.

Dinosaur Valley State Park was created in 1969 with a small but informative museum attached to the entrance station. Also, there is a gift store located just down the park road with enough dinosaur books, T-shirts, and other gift items to satisfy any parent's educational shopping list. If you have trouble finding the gift shop, just look for the two life-size fiberglass models of a 70-foot Brontosaurus and a 45-foot Tyrannosaurus rex, which were previously seen lurking around the 1964–1965 New York World's Fair. While your first impression may be that these large replicas belong in a Pee-wee Herman movie rather than a state park, they are a magnet for children and give adults a real sense of how monstrous these creatures really were.

Luckily for campers looking for quiet, the campgrounds are located away from the more heavily traveled areas. The first is North Primitive Camping Area, which is accessible only to backpackers willing to make the wet crossing of the Paluxy. The main camping area consists of 47 numbered spots, which have nice tree cover, are well spaced, and contain picnic tables, fireplaces, and a central bathroom/shower facility, but which unfortunately also allow RVs and trailers. While this would normally repel the tent-camping purist, the arrangement of the spaces with a central area of heavy trees makes it acceptable, especially to the first-time tent camper or a veteran bringing a load of inquisitive young dinosaur hunters.

Given the proximity to a large metropolitan area and its popularity with the fossil mania crowd, the campground can fill up quickly on weekends, so reservations are a must. As with most parks, the earlier you check in, the better your chances to get one of the riverside campsites 13–17. These sites are on a bluff backing up to the Paluxy, and normally allow a short hike to the river. Unfortunately, a series of heavy floods have made this access a little more difficult, ending with a 10-foot drop to the riverbed. Don't worry, however, as the other river access points are still intact, and a good pair of water shoes will make for easy crossing to the main hiking trails. These trails quickly take on a wilderness feel with nice lookouts over the river and surrounding parklands. It's always a good idea to view the park's website or Facebook page for current trail and river conditions.

When leaving the park on Park Road 59 (FM 205), don't miss the Fossil Rim Wildlife Center, located to the right on US 67. This first-class endangered species research and conservation complex features a drive-through experience among exotic animals, which are also part of a breeding program for endangered or threatened species, especially cheetahs. The best time to visit is in the morning when the animals are most active.

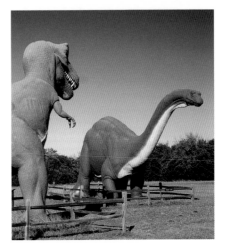

Probably not good tent buddies!

Turn left on US 67 to reach the town of Glen Rose. Travel into the town center to explore a traditional courthouse square surrounded by shops, and note the number of bed-and-breakfast options should the weather turn nasty or the dinosaur ghosts give your kids the spooks. This might happen especially around Halloween, a great time to visit Dinosaur Valley State Park.

VOICES FROM THE CAMPFIRE AND RECOMMENDED READING

Every father and mother here, if they are wise, will bring up their children not to shirk difficulties, but to meet them, and overcome them, not to strive after a life of ignoble ease, but to strive to do their duty, first to themselves and their families, and then to the whole state.
Theodore Roosevelt, *Strenuous Epigrams* (New York, H. M. Caldwell Co., 1904).

Unlike television, nature does not steal time; it amplifies it. Nature offers healing for a child living in a destructive family or neighborhood. It serves as a blank slate upon which a child draws and reinterprets the culture's fantasies. Nature inspires creativity in a child by demanding visualization and the full use of the senses. Given a chance, a child will bring the confusion of the world to the woods, wash it in the creek, turn it over to see what lives on the unseen side of that confusion. Nature can frighten a child, too, and this fright serves a purpose. In nature, a child finds freedom, fantasy, and privacy: a place distant from the adult world, a separate peace.
Richard Louv, *Last Child in the Woods* (Chapel Hill, NC, Algonquin Books of Chapel Hill, 2008).

BACKCOUNTRY ADVENTURES

As you turn off US 67 traveling toward the park, avert your eyes from the dinosaur tourist traps and enter the safe haven of the park. Park near the Cedar Brake trailhead and cross the Paluxy River if it is safe to do so. You may need water shoes if your hiking boots or walking shoes don't like too much to drink. Proceed up the bank and follow any of the trails by foot, or mountain bike where allowed. The views, especially from the scenic over-look, are great and a nearby large rock along the trail can provide a perfect place to stop for snacks. If you are tired and believe there is a shortcut down the hillside, think again before you find enough thorns and snakes to remind you to stay on trail. Of course, if a really large snake is sleeping in the sun across your trail, you may detour around it or better yet, go the other way.

BEST LOCAL FOOD AND DRINK

The Glen Rose area offers a number of locally owned restaurants, including Hammonds BBQ (254-897-3008; hammondsbbq.com), the Green Pickle (254-898-1611) for burgers, and Pie Peddlers (254-897-4904) and Shoo-Fly Soda Shop (254-396-0767) for a sweet treat. For a real Texas experience, get off the main road and feast at the Loco Coyote (254-897-2324; lococoyotegrill.com), about 15 minutes west of the park. Just don't go if you're in a hurry—it's a place to relax and enjoy!

Dinosaur Valley State Park

GETTING THERE

From Glen Rose, travel west on US 67 to Park Road 59 (FM 205) and turn right. At about 3 miles, stay to the right at the fork. The park entrance is 1 mile straight ahead.

GPS COORDINATES: N32° 14.826' W97° 48.894'

22

Eisenhower State Park: LAKE TEXOMA

Beauty: ★★★★ / Privacy: ★★★ / Spaciousness: ★★★ / Quiet: ★★★ / Security: ★★★★ / Cleanliness: ★★★

At 89,000 acres Lake Texoma has enough play space for all visitors.

It's not very often that Texans and Oklahomans can agree to share anything, but the massive 89,000-acre Lake Texoma that forms a large section of the border between the two states has enough play space for all visitors. The lake was formed in 1944 when the U.S. Army Corps of Engineers impounded the muddy Red River. Over the years, the lake has grown so large and deep that except during the wettest season, the lake water is clear and perfect for all forms of boating, from large sailboats and motor yachts to canoes and kayaks. The 580-mile shoreline provides enough hidden coves for some peace and quiet, except for the busiest of holidays in the summer. Just arrive on a weekday and have a local boat guide, a friend familiar with the lake, or a very good lake map. Yes, it really is that big.

After a long day of water sports, the tent camper will enjoy Eisenhower State Park, located on the southern Texas shore near the dam and spillway area. From the entrance station, travel Park Road 20 past the boat ramp, the boathouses, screened-in shelters, and the usual RV sites until you reach Fossil Ridge Campground turnoff at about 1.5 miles. Turn right for tent sites 144–165. These sites are heavily treed, and even though the terrain is rocky and hilly, the park has created some nice level tent sites. As you get nearer the water, sites 151–154 will give you a little lake view and easy access to a steep but good trail to a small fishing dock. From this dock or from your boat, you can angle for fish of all kinds, including striped bass, slab-sided crappie, and catfish big enough for the tallest tales around the campfire.

Returning to the main road, a short drive of 0.3 mile will take you past the showers/restrooms to Elm Point Camping Area. Follow the signs to sites 167–179 and enjoy the

Visit off-season for your own private beach.

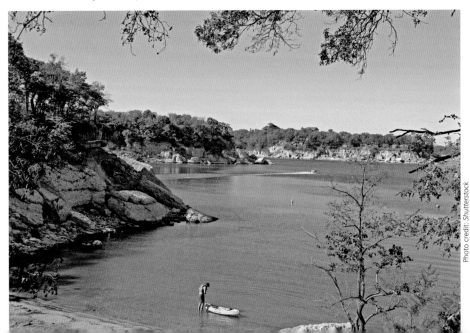

Photo credit: *Shutterstock*

KEY INFORMATION

ADDRESS: 50 Park Road 20, Denison, TX 75020-4878

CONTACT: 903-465-1956, tpwd.texas.gov/state-parks/eisenhower

OPERATED BY: Texas Parks & Wildlife Department

OPEN: Year-round

SITES: 190 (58 water only)

EACH SITE: Tent sites 144–190 have picnic tables, fire rings, water, and lantern hooks

ASSIGNMENT: First come, first served until site-specific reservation system begins in 2018

REGISTRATION: At headquarters or reserve at texas.reserveworld.com or 512-389-8900

FACILITIES: Restrooms and showers

PARKING: At each site

FEE: $17 premium sites 167–179, other tent sites $15, overflow sites $12; $5/person entrance fee, age 12 and under free

ELEVATION: 717'

RESTRICTIONS:

PETS: On leash only

FIRES: In fire rings only

ALCOHOL: Prohibited in all public/outdoor areas

VEHICLES: 2/site

OTHER: Maximum 8 people/site; guests must leave by 10 p.m.; quiet time 10 p.m.–6 a.m.; bring your own firewood or charcoal; limited supplies at park store; pick up main supplies in Denison or Sherman; gathering firewood prohibited

views from this peninsula perched high above lake level. Especially in summer, these sites will give you the best breeze while maintaining a nice tree cover of cedar elms and mature oaks. If you arrive early enough and have luck on your side, you can secure site 179, which offers a 180-degree view of the lake from the rocky point. Just be careful if you sleepwalk or go out for a night stroll. The cliffs are dangerous, and there are no guardrails for the careless or the intoxicated.

Heading back toward the entrance, you can visit the Eisenhower Yacht Club for boat rentals. In Denison, visit the childhood home of President Dwight D. Eisenhower, the park's namesake. Just west of Denison and its neighbor to the south, Sherman, travel west on US 82 to the Hagerman National Wildlife Refuge. This well-known but remote refuge is a popular stopover for migrating birds taking advantage of the Lake Texoma backwaters, ponds, and even cooperating farmers who grow "bird food" crops in the area.

VOICES FROM THE CAMPFIRE AND RECOMMENDED READING

We are all of us children of earth—grant us that simple knowledge. If our brothers are oppressed, then we are oppressed. If they hunger, we hunger. If their freedom is taken away, our freedom is not secure. Grant us a common faith that man shall know bread and peace, that he shall know justice and righteousness, freedom and security, an equal opportunity and an equal chance to do his best, not only in our own lands but throughout the world, and in that faith let us march toward the clean world our hands can make. Amen.

Donald Porter Geddes, ed., Franklin Delano Roosevelt: A Memorial (New York, Pocket Books, 1945).

Author's note: FDR recited this prayer in a radio address for Flag Day on June 14, 1942.

BACKCOUNTRY ADVENTURES

When you check in at the entrance station, the experienced and friendly staff will help you find the best ways to safely enjoy Lake Texoma. Unless you get a guide, a good lake map is essential, and all safety rules are strictly enforced on the lake. Ample mountain bike trails are located off the main park road. Once you leave the park and its peaceful setting, you can also go north on US 75 toward Durant to enjoy some casino games of chance, which are not allowed on the Texas side of the Red River.

BEST LOCAL FOOD AND DRINK

Denison is only a 15-minute drive from the park and has a surprising number of good local eateries. Try Huck's Catfish (903-337-0033; huckscatfish.com), Nick's Family Restaurant (903-463-3687), North Rig Grill for a Texas-size lunch (903-464-9999), the Old Mining Camp Smokehouse (903-463-0227), or Byrd & Mike's (903-337-1722; chestnutstreetpub .com) to enjoy tasty food and beer in a beer garden on a hot day.

Eisenhower State Park: Lake Texoma

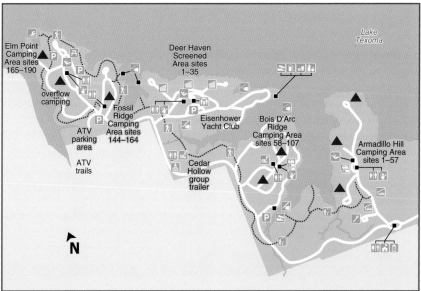

GETTING THERE

Take US 75 north from Dallas approximately 75 miles. Go past Sherman, and just north of Denison, exit onto TX 91. Turn left. The park entrance is 4 miles straight ahead.

GPS COORDINATES: N33° 48.618' W96° 36.000'

23

Lake Mineral Wells State Park & Trailway

Beauty: ★★★ / Privacy: ★★★ / Spaciousness: ★★★ / Quiet: ★★ / Security: ★★★★ / Cleanliness: ★★★

Check out more than 22 miles of mountain biking, hiking, and equestrian trails from Lake Mineral Wells Trailway trailhead.

Located 1 hour west of Fort Worth, the gateway to the wide-open spaces of West Texas, this park has the advantage of being at the northern edge of Texas Hill Country, and most important, of a 670-acre lake. After leaving the entrance station, the park road reaches an overlook of the lake. A left turn at 0.5 mile will take you to a protected sandy beach area and the park store, which also serves as the rental center for canoes and kayaks. The camping supplies are limited, but the store stocks a good selection of emergency ice cream and cold drinks. Leaving the parking lot, turn left and look for the Lake Mineral Wells Trailway trailhead at 1 mile. This is your connection to more than 22 miles of mountain biking, hiking, and equestrian trails. Leaving the trailhead parking lot, turn right for a 0.6-mile scenic drive with access to multiple picnic tables high on a bluff overlooking the lake. At the end of the road, park at Penitentiary Hollow and descend the short but narrow trail into the heart of a large boulder field, where local climbers practice their moves. However, don't be fooled by a lack of alpine vistas—a slip of the hand without proper protection can shatter an ankle in a split second.

Returning to the park store/beach area, the spillway turnoff is immediately on your right and serves as the only access to the camping area. The first right at 0.4 mile is for screened shelters 1–15. The sites run $36 per day and have sufficient space for extra tents. They're

Lake Mineral Wells Trailway is a must-visit for hikers and bikers.

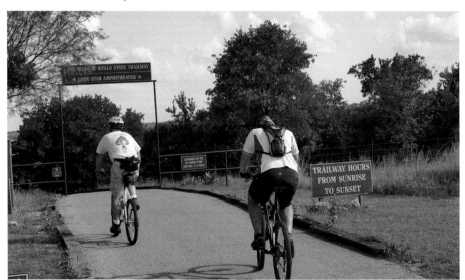

KEY INFORMATION

ADDRESS: 100 Park Road 71,
Mineral Wells, TX 76067

CONTACT: 940-328-1171, tpwd.texas.gov
/state-parks/lake-mineral-wells

OPERATED BY: Texas Parks & Wildlife
Department

OPEN: Year-round

SITES: 108 (31 water only: 20 in Cross
Timbers, 11 in Post Oak)

EACH SITE: Water, picnic table, fire ring,
lantern pole

ASSIGNMENT: First come, first served
until site-specific reservation system
begins in 2018

REGISTRATION: At headquarters or reserve
at texas.reserveworld.com or
512-389-8900

FACILITIES: Showers at all campgrounds

except Post Oak; centrally located
flush toilets

PARKING: At each site

FEE: $14/water-only tent site; $7/person
entrance fee, age 12 and under free;
$3 for rock climbing

ELEVATION: 539'

RESTRICTIONS:

PETS: On leash only

FIRES: In fire rings or grates only

ALCOHOL: Prohibited in all public/
outdoor areas

VEHICLES: 2/site

OTHER: Maximum 8 people/site; guests must
leave by 10 p.m.; quiet time 10 p.m.–
6 a.m.; bring your own firewood or
charcoal; limited supplies at park store;
pick up main supplies in Mineral Wells;
gathering firewood prohibited

situated on a nice bluff overlooking the lake. Back on the main road, turn left at 0.4 mile for the Cross Timbers Camping Area and sites 89–108. This water-only area affords some peace and quiet from the electrified RV areas, and it also accesses the 12-mile Cross Timbers Back Country Trail, which allows hiking, mountain biking, and equestrian use. The central parking lot located at the entrance to the campsite road is also the trailhead for the 2.5-mile Primitive Campground Access Trail for the backpackers in your group looking to pitch their tents away from any motorized, two-wheeled, or four-legged neighbors. Cross Timbers Campground has showers and bathrooms near site 90, and the heavy tree cover of post oaks, blackjack oaks, and cedar elm provide some privacy and welcome shade.

Returning to the main road, turn left and take an immediate right into Post Oak Camping Area for tent sites 1–11. This hilly, rocky, and tree-covered campground runs along the ridge with a lake view. There are no showers, but the small number of sites will give you a more remote feeling, and the lake breeze is a lifesaver in summer.

When leaving the park, be sure to turn right to visit the town of Mineral Wells. This community became famous in the late 1800s when the natural mineral springs became a mecca for tourists seeking the medicinal properties of these healing waters. As you head east back toward Fort Worth, watch for the sign to Clark Gardens (940-682-4856; clarkgardens.org) at about 3 miles. It's a true oasis in this mostly dry West Texas locale. In summer, don't miss the Parker County peaches in Weatherford before returning to the big-city bustle of Fort Worth.

VOICES FROM THE CAMPFIRE AND RECOMMENDED READING

I would never betray a friend to serve a cause. Never reject a friend to help an institution. Great nations may fall in ruin before I would sell a friend to save them.
Edward Abbey, *A Voice Crying in the Wilderness* (New York, St. Martin's Press, 1989).

BACKCOUNTRY ADVENTURES

While the areas in Texas that have the right geology for rock climbing or bouldering are limited, the Penitentiary Hollow is an excellent place for adventure if you have the skills and experience. Watching the climbers will give you a good idea that this is not for the novice without proper training. Attempting a climb or a repel will give you a very small taste of big wall climbs in Yosemite, Zion, or the Grand Tetons. For a less dangerous adventure, the Lake Mineral Wells Trailway system will give you a great workout whether by bike, hike, or horse.

BEST LOCAL FOOD AND DRINK

For a home-cooked, hearty breakfast to fill up on before a morning hike, drive a few blocks south of downtown to Jimmy's Cafe (940-325-9997). Pick up a healthy lunch to go from Brazos Market & Bistro (940-468-2702; brazosmarket.com), or reward yourself after a long morning ride with lunch and homemade dessert at the Black Horse Café (940-325-8787), whose offerings include great panini and a daily Italian special (I hear the lasagna is amazing!). The Mesquite Pit (940-325-5960; mesquitepit.com) is a local go-to spot for steak or brisket at lunch on Sundays, or anytime the rest of the week.

Lake Mineral Wells State Park & Trailway

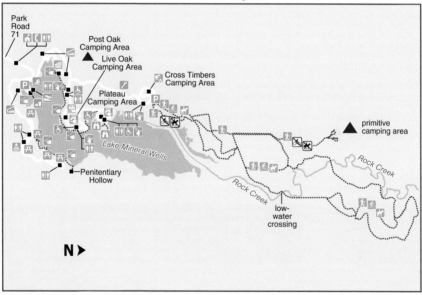

GETTING THERE

From Fort Worth, travel 20 miles west on I-20, and exit onto US 180 at Weatherford. Travel 18 miles through Weatherford toward Mineral Wells. Turn right onto Park Road 71, and the entrance to the park is 2.7 miles straight ahead.

GPS COORDINATES: N32° 48.786' W98° 2.586'

24

Lyndon B. Johnson National Grasslands

Beauty: ★★★ / Privacy: ★★ / Spaciousness: ★★★ / Quiet: ★★★ / Security: ★★ / Cleanliness: ★★★

Slow down, open your windows, and keep a sharp watch for bobcats.

When planning your next tent-camping trip, the Lyndon B. Johnson National Grasslands is a nice surprise. While the name conjures visions of mile after mile of treeless expanse, the area is actually a huge park of trees, lakes, and rolling hills. The trail system covers more than 75 miles.

The initial approach from the highway gives the appearance of modern ranchette civilization, but that quickly gives way after you turn onto County Road 2461, 0.5 mile from Black Creek Lake Campground. Be sure to slow down, open your windows, and keep a sharp watch for bobcats or other animals crossing the road. A sign ahead will direct you to the final 0.5-mile stretch to the Black Creek campground and lake area, which is surrounded by towering pines and oaks. The central parking area contains the self-registration drop ("fee tube"), a concrete boat ramp, and the central vault toilet. The area contains 11 campsites. Vehicles are restricted to the parking area.

Many tent campers used to head across the lake to the scenic sites by the shore, but the wooden bridge is gone and that area has been decommissioned. Instead, take time for a stroll into the backwoods area, where you will have a good chance to meet white-tailed deer, coyotes, and red and gray fox, along with various birds, such as quail and wild turkeys. Black Creek does not allow horses or hunting, so it should be quiet and rewarding.

Leaving the parking area, return to the main road, turn left, and follow the signs to TADRA Point. The road is well-maintained gravel, but watch your speed: the wild turkeys that also use this road seem rather surprised to hear a vehicle in their territory. In 1.1 miles, turn left onto FS 904. In another 0.8 mile, turn right onto FS 900, and turn left into TADRA

A quiet stroll with the local wildlife will be your best reward.

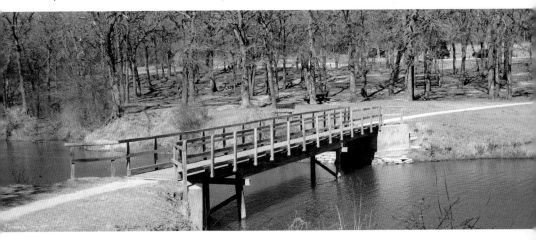

KEY INFORMATION

ADDRESS: 1400 N. US 287,
Decatur, Texas 76234

OPERATED BY: U.S. Forest Service

CONTACT: 940-627-5475,
tinyurl.com/lbjnatlgrass

OPEN: Year-round

SITES: Black Creek Lake: 11 walk-in with
picnic table; TADRA: number of sites varies,
no tables; Valley View: 11 in grassy area;
group site; call for availability and
permit information

EACH SITE: Fire ring

ASSIGNMENT: First come, first served

REGISTRATION: Drop box at entrance area
to each campground

FACILITIES: Vault toilets; no water
or electricity

PARKING: Central parking at Black Creek
Lake; parking at sites in TADRA

FEE: Black Creek Lake: $2/night or day use;
TADRA: $4/night or day use

ELEVATION: 967'

RESTRICTIONS:

PETS: On leash only

FIRES: In fire rings only (check for fire
danger level)

ALCOHOL: Prohibited

VEHICLES: 2/site

OTHER: Maximum 8 people/site; guests must
leave by 10 p.m.; quiet time 10 p.m.–6
a.m.; bring your own firewood or charcoal;
pick up main supplies in Decatur; gathering
firewood allowed from downed wood only

Point at 0.9 mile. There is a covered pavilion for group events, and the sites provide drive-in convenience along with vault toilets. This large campground contains a network of 20 parking spurs and 6 pull-throughs for vehicles with horse trailers. The tree cover is nice, and sites are separated by heavy brush. Some sites sit on a slight downhill slope, but these are also the most remote.

The central road is dirt with gravel and also functions as a horse trail, which is part of a 75-mile trail system for horses, hikers, and mountain bikers. All trails are multiuse. All horses must have their Coggins certification prior to heading out.

The TADRA Point trailhead functions as the confluence for the trail system. Local equestrian groups, whose volunteer labor created the extensive options into the backcountry, use this system. A good sign of remoteness is the bulletin board instructions labeled WHAT IF I GET LOST? As a final note, remember to check with the Grasslands headquarters about fire danger and what areas might be open to hunting. Of course, if you are combining tent camping and hunting, then security will probably not be a big concern in this rough, backwoods area of North Texas. No matter what activity you enjoy, the rough terrain and the sight of Texans on horseback will be a vivid reminder of the bygone era of cattle drives, when nearly 10 million cattle and their escorts traveled north to markets over these vast grasslands.

VOICES FROM THE CAMPFIRE AND RECOMMENDED READING

Had the Indian and not the white man written history, he would have filled it with true stories of the hazardous feats of warriors in carrying their slain or wounded comrades off the field of battle.

Walter Prescott Webb, *The Texas Rangers: A Century of Frontier Defense* (Boston, Houghton Mifflin Company, 1935).

BACKCOUNTRY ADVENTURES

This U.S. Forest Service area is a mecca for the equestrian crowd, and it has enough open space for you to feel like a pioneer arriving from points north and east. Only a century or so ago, you would not be surprised if a covered wagon came over the hill on these rutted dirt and rock roads, bringing new settlers to the North Texas area but still wary of crossing into Kiowa or Comanche territory.

BEST LOCAL FOOD AND DRINK

If it's convenient with your travel plans, skip the usual chain restaurants along US 287 and enjoy local establishments around the Decatur town square, including top-rated Sweetie Pie's Ribeyes (940-626-4555; sweetiepiesribeyes.com) or a brisket burger at Rooster's Roadhouse (940-626-8044; roosters-roadhouse.com).

Lyndon B. Johnson National Grasslands

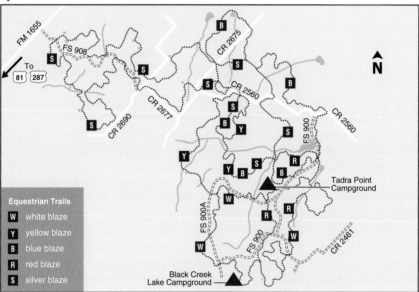

GETTING THERE

From the intersection of US 380 and US 287 in Decatur, travel 0.5 mile north on US 287 to the LBJ National Grasslands District Office. Continue 3.3 miles farther north to County Road 2175. Make a hard-right turn and follow the signs 11.2 miles to Black Creek Lake. See the profile above for directions from Black Creek Lake Campground to TADRA Campground.

GPS COORDINATES: N33° 20.682' W97° 35.682'

25

Possum Kingdom State Park

Beauty: ★★★★ / Privacy: ★★★ / Spaciousness: ★★★ / Quiet: ★★★ / Security: ★★★ / Cleanliness: ★★★

Enjoy beautiful lake views and your own private trail down to the water's edge.

As you leave Mineral Wells heading west on US 180, you cross the legendary Brazos River and head into Hill Country beauty known as the Palo Pinto Mountains. The wide vistas and juniper-covered hills are dotted with longhorn cattle, pumping oil wells, cacti, and windmills that give this remote area a special place in Texas history. It is still sparsely populated and only a tough breed of Texan chooses to work and live in these rugged hills.

After passing Caddo, turn right on Park Road 33 and follow the winding paved road for 15 miles until the park entrance sign. Go straight ahead for 0.4 mile and stop at the historical marker on your left that details the hard work of the Civilian Conservation Corps (CCC) sent here in May 1941 to build the park's infrastructure. As the Second World War began taking in large numbers of recruits, this CCC camp was the last one closed in July 1942. Accustomed to military-type discipline and outdoor experiences, these previously unemployed men were perfect candidates to become the Greatest Generation.

Continuing past the entrance station for 0.3 mile, turn right on PR 33, following the signs toward campsites 22–116. Twenty-thousand-acre Possum Kingdom Lake appears on

A lakeside picnic will soothe your soul.

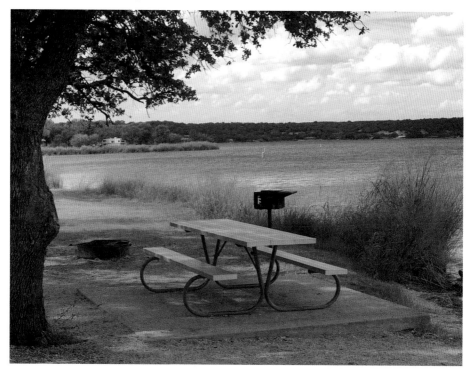

KEY INFORMATION

ADDRESS: 3901 State Park Road 33, Caddo, TX 76429

CONTACT: 940-549-1803, tpwd.texas.gov /state-parks/possum-kingdom

OPERATED BY: Texas Parks & Wildlife Department

OPEN: Year-round

SITES: 15 at Lakeview, 37 at Chaparral Trail

EACH SITE: Picnic table, fire ring, upright grate

ASSIGNMENT: First come, first served until site-specific reservation system begins in 2018

REGISTRATION: At headquarters or reserve at texas.reserveworld.com or 512-389-8900

FACILITIES: Modern restrooms and showers, park store, canoe and kayak rentals

PARKING: At each site

FEE: $7 primitive walk-in, $12 water-only; $4/person entrance fee, under 13 free

ELEVATION: 1,033'

RESTRICTIONS:

PETS: On leash only

FIRES: In fire rings or grates only

ALCOHOL: Prohibited in all public/ outdoor areas

VEHICLES: 2/site

OTHER: No potable water in park for drinking or cooking as of publication date; non-potable water suitable for bathing, washing, and cleaning is available at campsites, restrooms, and showers; maximum 8 people/ site; guests must leave by 10 p.m.; quiet time 10 p.m.–6 a.m.; bring your own firewood or charcoal; limited supplies at park store; pick up main supplies in Mineral Wells or Breckenridge; gathering firewood prohibited

your left through the junipers, and the primitive sites are on the left at lake level. These sites are adequate but probably better as overflow sites. The first numbered sites begin on the left with sites 22–25 on the water. Site 26 is the premium waterfront site, where you can hear the waves from your tent. While there is also a huge shade tree with a small sandy beach,

Covered tables, great views . . . tent camping at its best.

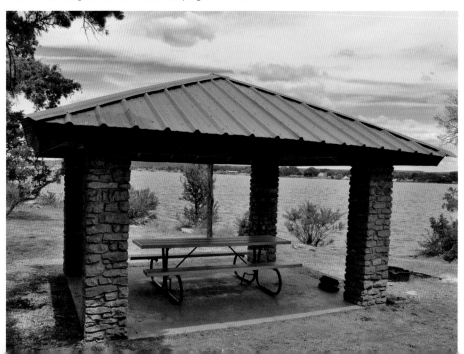

make sure your tent and camping gear are anchored down, since a stiff lake breeze could easily send your lightweight items in for an unplanned swim.

Returning to the main road, turn right at the boat ramp, proceed past the restrooms and showers, and pass straight through the Shady Grove RV camping area. As you enter the Chaparral camping area, you begin with sites 79–81 on the left and a selection of some of the best tent campsites in Texas. With covered picnic tables and elevated views of Possum Kingdom Lake, these popular overnight spots fill up quickly.

Proceeding on, the main road splits to the right along interior sites 86–99. Beginning with site 100, the lake comes back into view with your own private trail down to the water's edge. Sites 101–116 continue along the rocky cliff, providing premier camping with commanding lake views and a wilderness feel. Look for site 113 for the highest point in the campground.

Returning to the main road, turn right toward the park store and marina. Rental boats are available, as well as a protected swimming area and 2.5 miles of hiking trails. Also, don't miss the wide range of birds, including hawks, herons, hummingbirds, and turkey vultures. Finally, as you close the tent fly for the night, look for the park's namesake, the opossum.

VOICES FROM THE CAMPFIRE AND RECOMMENDED READING

In that place the stark pleasures of aloneness and unchangingness and what a river meant did not somehow seem to be very explicable. . . . You are not in a hurry there; you learned long since not to be.

John Graves, *Goodbye to a River* (Philadelphia, The Curtis Publishing Company, 1959).

Author's note: John Graves took a farewell canoe trip down the Brazos River in Texas before it was dammed and changed forever.

I thrive best on solitude. If I have had a companion only one day in a week, unless it were one or two I could name, I find that the value of the week to me has been seriously affected. It dissipates my days, and often it takes me another week to get over it.

Henry David Thoreau, *The Journal of Henry David Thoreau, 1837-1861* (New York, New York Review Books Classics, 2009).

The study of the relationship between mental acuity, creativity, and time spent outdoors is a frontier for science. But new research suggests that exposure to the living world can enhance intelligence for some people. This probably happens in at least two ways: first, our senses and sensibilities are improved through our direct interaction with nature (and practical knowledge of natural systems is still applicable in our everyday lives); second, a more natural environment seems to stimulate our ability to pay attention, think clearly, and be more creative, even in dense urban neighborhoods. This research has positive implications for education, for business, and for the daily lives of young and old.

Richard Louv, *The Nature Principle: Reconnecting with Life in a Virtual Age* (Chapel Hill, NC, Algonquin Books of Chapel Hill, 2012).

BACKCOUNTRY ADVENTURES

The sheer size and great water quality of Possum Kingdom Lake make any water sport here a joy. At sunset, the towering rock cliffs along its 310 miles of shoreline are reason enough to just float anywhere you want. In the future, look for Texas's newest state park located just west of Strawn. When open to the public, Palo Pinto Mountains State Park will offer rugged terrain for not only adventure, but also easy access to Mary's Cafe, in case your cookstove runs out of fuel.

BEST LOCAL FOOD AND DRINK

On your way to the park, stop at Mary's Cafe (254-672-5741) in Strawn for its famous chicken-fried steak. (Fill your gas tank too.) If you can't wait for Mary's Cafe, try New York Hill Restaurant (254-672-5848; thurbernewyorkhill.com) in Mingus or 526 Pizza Studio (940-549-6606; tastingsgrahamtx.com) in Graham, which offers amazing gluten-free choices. The park store has basic supplies, and the owner Jeff is a wealth of information when it comes to the park and nearby amenities.

Possum Kingdom State Park

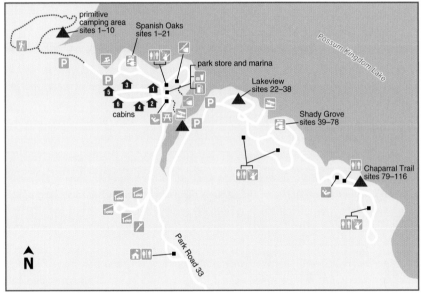

GETTING THERE

From Mineral Wells, drive 35.5 miles west on US 180. Turn right onto PR 33 and drive 17 miles north to the park entrance.

GPS COORDINATES: N32° 52.608' W98° 33.696'

Purtis Creek State Park

Beauty: ★★★ / Privacy: ★★★ / Spaciousness: ★★★ / Quiet: ★★★★ / Security: ★★★★ / Cleanliness: ★★★

Sample the pleasures of fishing, bird-watching, and quiet boating while enjoying the shade of massive oaks and junipers in this family-friendly park.

Located along US 175 and near the gateway to heavily treed East Texas, Purtis Creek State Park is a prime fishing lake. The 355-acre lake was built to control floodwaters but has become a first-class destination for anglers who don't want to fight the speedboat crowd. There is a 50-boat limit on the lake, and the no-wake rule is strictly enforced, with a speed limit appropriately described as "idle."

Turning north off US 175, you'll approach the park past tranquil farms and small ranches. After leaving the headquarters, you'll see the lake almost immediately, with sites 60–64 straight ahead near the boat docks and protected swimming area. These sites are perfect for families out for a weekend of water fun, but those looking for solitude should proceed to the primitive campground parking lot and take the short nature trail to sites A through M. After leaving your car, follow the easy dirt trail across two small wooden bridges and then to a fork. The left fork takes you to the chemical toilet. The right fork crosses the third wooden bridge. About 5 minutes later, you'll arrive at a nicely constructed bird-watcher's

You can paddle your canoe or kayak right up to your doorstep.

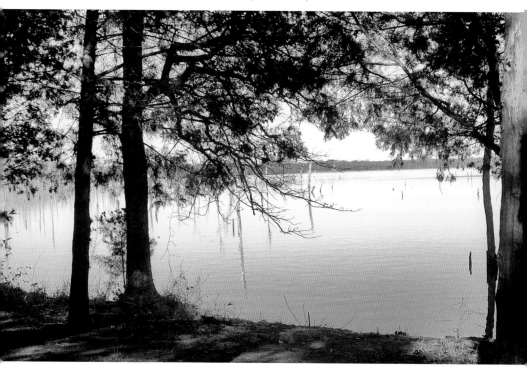

KEY INFORMATION

ADDRESS: 14225 FM 316,
Eustace, TX 75124

CONTACT: 903-425-2332,
tpwd.texas.gov/state-parks/purtis-creek

OPERATED BY: Texas Parks & Wildlife
Department

OPEN: Year-round

SITES: 18

EACH SITE: Sites A–M, fire rings; sites
60–64, water taps; picnic tables and
bathrooms nearby

ASSIGNMENT: First come, first served
until site-specific reservation system
begins in 2018

REGISTRATION: At headquarters or reserve
at texas.reserveworld.com or
512-389-8900

FACILITIES: Bathrooms and showers at
multiuse camping area

PARKING: Small paved lot near trailhead
(sites A–M); at sites 60–64

FEE: $10 primitive sites (A–M), $14 water-
only sites (60–64); $5/person entrance fee,
age 12 and under free

ELEVATION: 374'

RESTRICTIONS:

PETS: On leash only

FIRES: In fire rings only; firewood is $3/stack
at host site 16

ALCOHOL: Prohibited in all public/
outdoor areas

VEHICLES: 2/site

OTHER: Maximum 8 people/site; guests must
leave by 10 p.m.; quiet time 10 p.m.–
6 a.m.; bring your own firewood or
charcoal; limited supplies in Eustace;
main supplies in Kaufman or Athens

blind complete with an opening for cameras or binoculars. The trail continues along the edge of this very quiet backwater area until you reach sites A through M in about another 5 minutes. These nicely spaced sites are primitive, but they have the advantage of privacy and waterfront views for the more than 200 bird species that call this park home at different times of the year. However, the most unique feature is the ability to pull your boat up to a smooth landing and deliver your camping gear by boat rather than pack it in by the trail. Call the park or check their website to see if canoe rentals are available.

This area was also home to the Wichita and Caddo tribes who left petroglyphs just east of the park, indicating this land was also good for hunting. As the frontier was explored and conquered, the conflict between American Indians and white settlers flared and resulted in the death of famed Cherokee Indian Chief Bowles, who was slain in the Battle of Neches in 1839 near the town of Edom.

For the tent camper today, it is easy to see the attraction for all those who have passed here before. The abundant wildlife, rich vegetation, and clean water were vital to survival then and provide a perfect escape from the clogged freeways of the big city today. While the bass fishing is world-class, don't miss the many canoeing activities, including classes in basic canoe skills and even a Full Moon Canoe Tour. Canoeing or kayaking this peaceful area provides the serenity and relaxation you can only get from calm water. Whatever your interest, don't miss this hidden gem that's a little more than an hour away from Dallas.

VOICES FROM THE CAMPFIRE AND RECOMMENDED READING

Letter of Chief Seathl (Seattle) of the Suwamish Tribe to the President of the United States of America, Franklin Pierce, 1854

The Great Chief in Washington sends word that he wishes to buy our land. The Great Chief also sends us words of friendship and good will. This is kind of him, since we know he has little need of our friendship in return. But we will consider your offer. For we know that if we do not sell, the white man may come with guns and take our land.

How can you buy or sell the sky, the warmth of the land? The idea is strange to us. If we do not own the freshness of the air and the sparkle of the water, how can you buy them?

Every part of this earth is sacred to my people. Every shining pine needle, every sandy shore, every mist in the dark woods, every clearing, and every humming insect is holy in the memory and experience of my people. The sap which courses through the trees carries the memories of the red man. So, when the Great Chief in Washington sends word that he wishes to buy our land, he asks much of us.

Ed McGaa, Eagle Man, Mother Earth Spirituality (New York, HarperCollins, 1990).

BACKCOUNTRY ADVENTURES

If available, rent a kayak, canoe, or paddleboat from the park store, or bring your own and enjoy time viewing all parts of this quiet lake, known for its exceptional bass fishing and bird-watching. Drive to the trailhead if you must, or better yet, park near the park store, throw your gear in a canoe, and paddle across the lake to the primitive campsites. Beaver Slide Nature Path is a pleasant, mostly shaded, easy 1.7-mile loop trail, where adventurers of all ages can search for animal tracks and watch for turtles sunning themselves on logs along the inlet.

BEST LOCAL FOOD AND DRINK

On summer weekends, watch for an old-fashioned shaved ice stand on the north side of US 175 while going through Eustace. If you're hungry for more than dessert and driving

Purtis Creek may be close to the big city, but it feels light years away.

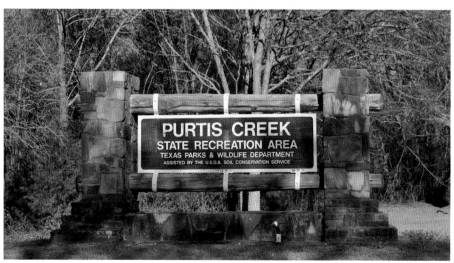

north on US 175, in Kemp try El Manantial for Mexican dishes (903-432-1234) or Milano's Pizza (903-432-9199; milanospizzatx.com). If driving west, in Seven Points you might try Cedar Creek Brewery (903-432-2337; cedarcreekbrewery.com), Molly's Catfish Corner (903-432-3445; mollyscatfishcorner.com), or Tavi's Italian Restaurant (903-432-0330; facebook.com/TavisRestaurant). While part of a Texas-based chain, Dairy Queen restaurants (903-887-8361; dairyqueen.com) are a staple for any tent camper on a road trip, including in the Mabank area. If traveling near Athens, get a healthy start with a box of Daylight Donuts (903-675-2968; daylightdonuts.com), or have lunch at Railway Cafe (903-264-7245; railwaycafe.net) or the Jalapeno Tree (903-677-4056; jalapenotree.com).

Purtis Creek State Park

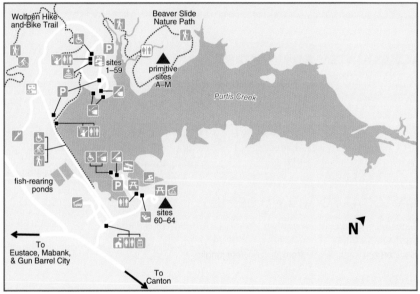

GETTING THERE

From US 175 between Kaufman and Athens, travel north on FM 316 for 3.3 miles to the park entrance on the left.

GPS COORDINATES: N32° 21.834' W96° 0.168'

27

Ray Roberts Lake State Park:

ISLE DU BOIS UNIT AND JOHNSON BRANCH

Beauty: ★★★ / Privacy: ★★★★ / Spaciousness: ★★★★ / Quiet: ★★★ / Security: ★★★★ / Cleanliness: ★★★★

As an urban escape, any time is a great time to visit.

There is something attractive about large bodies of water, especially when they are less than 1.5 hours from the urban sprawl of Dallas–Fort Worth. Located just north of the college town of Denton, Lake Ray Roberts is a 30,000-surface-acre reservoir with an irregular shoreline, which creates numerous peninsulas, backwater coves, and a sense of wildness not found in many man-made bodies of water. The large expanses of water serve as perfect sunrise and sunset reflectors as well as a summer playground for the powerboat set, which tells you that the best times to tent-camp here are during the week or anytime from late September to early May. Of course, this also corresponds with the best time to tent-camp in North Texas, since daytime summer temperatures here are often over 100°F and nighttime temperatures may not drop below 80°F. However, the presence of the lake will also give you a refreshing breeze and a protected swimming area in a small cove. Given this park's proximity as an urban escape, anytime is a great time to visit.

Turning north off FM 455, the headquarters and entrance station of the Isle du Bois Unit is 0.4 mile ahead. After paying your fees and picking up the park map, proceed past the small interpretive center and travel 1.5 miles to the Hawthorn Camping Area and turn left. The large paved parking lot and modern restrooms may not look like the access point

This waterfront gem isn't far from the concrete jungle.

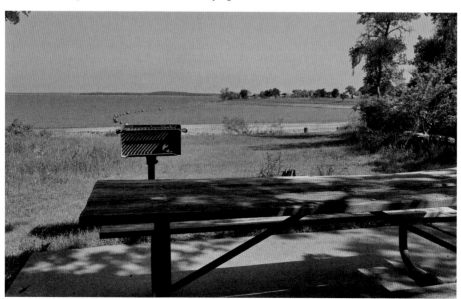

KEY INFORMATION

ADDRESS: Isle du Bois Unit: 100 PW 4137, Pilot Point, TX 76258; **Johnson Branch:** 100 PW 4153, Valley View, TX 76272

CONTACT: 940-686-2148 (Isle de Bois), 940 637-2294 (Johnson), tpwd.texas.gov /state-parks/ray-roberts-lake

OPERATED BY: Texas Parks & Wildlife Department

OPEN: Year-round

SITES: 53 sites, 2 group sites (Isle du Bois); 70 (Johnson Branch)

EACH SITE: Picnic table, fire ring with grate

ASSIGNMENT: First come, first served until site-specific reservation system begins in 2018

REGISTRATION: At headquarters or reserve at texas.reserveworld.com or 512-389-8900

FACILITIES: Restroom at Hawthorn Area lot, chemical toilet at Wild Plum Area, showers at ramp and RV areas

PARKING: Central paved lot for tent sites

FEE: $15 tent sites; $30 group site (24 person max); $7/person entrance fee

ELEVATION: 651'

RESTRICTIONS:

PETS: On leash only

FIRES: Check with headquarters; stoves OK

ALCOHOL: Prohibited in all public/ outdoor areas

VEHICLES: 2/site

OTHER: Maximum 8 people/site; guests must leave by 10 p.m.; quiet time 10 p.m.– 6 a.m.; bring your own firewood or charcoal; no park store; pick up main supplies in Sanger or Denton

to a wilderness tent-camping experience, but the best is hidden from immediate view. On your left, near the restrooms, are paved trails that lead to sites 6, 7, and 17, which are perfect for wheelchair access or other campers not able to walk to the wooded areas immediately behind these close-in sites.

As you proceed on the paved trail, it quickly gives way to a mostly gravel pathway, which is suitable for easy hiking to transport your camping gear to sites 8–15. As you walk, the stands of oak and elm become thicker and the sites get further apart. By the time you see the water, sites 10, 11, 13, 14, and 15 will give you waterfront views, and the parking lot will not be visible, even though the walk will have been less than 15 minutes.

If these sites are full or don't suit your desires, return to the parking lot and proceed to the end, where a similar set of close-in sites (18–21) would probably be acceptable, if you are not camping on a crowded weekend. However, continue into the woods and follow the trail until it splits at the directional sign. Sites 22–28 are to the right, but the better choice is to the left, where sites 29–34 will give you the camping experience of a more remote park. These sites follow the shoreline and are spaced to give you privacy and solitude. Sites 34A and 34B are especially nice for families who want the kids close by but not too close. Sites 27 and 29 are group sites that give excellent views of the lake, but are the farthest from the parking lot at about 20 minutes. The more you are able or willing to walk, the more secluded the sites become; these walks would even make for a good beginner backpack experience.

Leaving the Hawthorn Camping Area, turn left and travel for 0.7 mile until you see the Wild Plum Area parking lot on your left. Take the paved bicycle path for about 50 yards until you see the Wild Plum sign. The chemical toilets and campsites begin in about 75 yards. These sites (117–131) are in a nice grove of oak trees and are very close to a backwater cove; however, they also overlook the very large paved boat ramp area. While some park visitors would find it desirable to be near this very busy spot in the summer, the tent camper looking for some peace and quiet should return to Hawthorn, hike a little extra distance, and listen to the abundant bird life—including songbirds like cardinals and soaring red-tailed hawks being chased by local grackles.

After leaving Isle du Bois, return to I-35 North, take Exit 483, and travel 7 miles east on FM 3002 to the north shore of 30,000-acre Lake Ray Roberts, where the Johnson Branch provides the tent camper two totally different experiences. Just 0.4 mile after the entrance station, turn right into the Dogwood Canyon central parking area. From this location, you can unload your mountain bike and test your skills on nearly 9 miles of trails rated for different levels of expertise and used by the Dallas Off-Road Bicycle Association (dorba.org).

After a hard day on the bike, return to the parking lot and follow the dirt trail toward the lake and campsites 135–154. Look for sites 149 and 150 with waterfront access and views on a quiet backwater slough suitable for canoeing, kayaking, or a little fishing. The area is heavily wooded and the sites are spaced for privacy.

If you are looking for more of a lake experience, return to the park road, turn right, go past the RV campgrounds for 1.5 miles, and arrive at Oak Point. This large area contains the park store, picnic areas, boat ramps, modern restrooms, and showers, and a 180-degree view of the lake. The central parking for tent sites 106–134 is on your right, and a short walk will give you a great view and all the cool lake breezes you need. On busy weekends, there are also three overflow campgrounds with 25 additional sites. Look for 9 sites in overflow area C. These sites are right on the water and have covered picnic tables as well as a view of all the lake action, including windsurfers and parasailing.

Note: Some campsites may be slightly altered and/or sections of trails may be closed due to previous flooding. Contact the park for updates.

If you are bringing the family or need a place to float in peace, there is also a wide sandy beach with a protected swimming area. It is located behind the restrooms and overflow campsite A. Just follow the campers, hikers, bikers, and swimmers as they tow their ice chests to this popular area. There is no longer a park store, so bring your supplies with you or pick them up before arriving to explore this large lake, which is located less than 1.5 hours from Dallas or Fort Worth.

VOICES FROM THE CAMPFIRE AND RECOMMENDED READING

I shall look from the same window on the pure sea-green Walden water there, reflecting the clouds and the trees, and sending up its evaporations in solitude, and no traces will appear that a man has ever stood there.

Henry David Thoreau, *Walden, or Life in the Woods* (Boston, Ticknor and Fields, 1854).

We have yet to fully realize, or even adequately study, the enhancement of human capacities through the power of nature. . . . In fact, because of the environmental challenges we face today, we may be—we had better be—entering the most creative period in human history, a time defined by a goal that builds on and extends a century of environmentalism, which includes but goes beyond sustainability to the re-naturing of everyday life.

Richard Louv, *The Nature Principle: Reconnecting with Life in a Virtual Age* (Chapel Hill, NC, Algonquin Books of Chapel Hill, 2012).

BACKCOUNTRY ADVENTURES

The DORBA mountain biking trails are sufficient challenge for all skill levels, and equestrian camping is popular in this heart-of-Texas horse country.

BEST LOCAL FOOD AND DRINK

Before heading north out of Denton, load up on the best sandwiches at New York Sub-Way (940-566-1823) on US 380. Mexican food lovers will find multiple choices, including El Matador Restaurant (940-387-1137; elmatadorrestaurant.com) just off US 380 or Miguelito's (940-458-0073) in Sanger off I-35. Also enjoyable in Sanger is Babe's Chicken Dinner House (940-458-0000; babeschicken.com).

Ray Roberts Lake State Park: Isle du Bois Unit and Johnson Branch

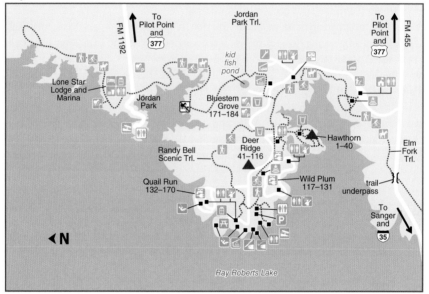

GETTING THERE

ISLE DU BOIS: From I-35, north of Denton, exit at Sanger. Take FM 455 east about 10 miles to the park entrance. From Pilot Point and US 377, take FM 455 west to the entrance.

    JOHNSON BRANCH: Take I-35 north from Dallas or Fort Worth. Go past Denton and take Exit 483. Go east on FM 3002 for 7 miles. Park entrance is on the right.

GPS COORDINATES:
    ISLE DU BOIS: N33° 21.907' W97° 0.845'
    JOHNSON BRANCH: N33° 25.781' W97° 3.388'

SOUTH TEXAS AND THE GULF COAST

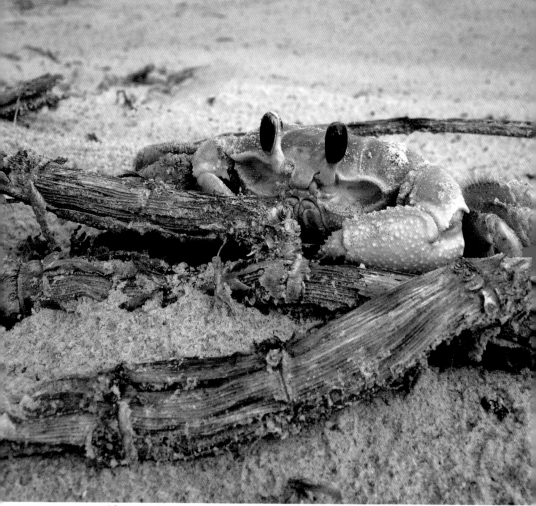

No need for a tent for this camper (Padre Island National Seashore; see page 122)

28

⛺ Brazos Bend State Park

Beauty: ★★★★ / Privacy: ★★★ / Spaciousness: ★★★ / Quiet: ★★★ / Security: ★★★★ / Cleanliness: ★★★

This special park will take you deep into our early history as Texans and even further.

When you are ready to escape the crowded confines of the big city, this special park will take you deep into our early history as Texans and even further—a lot further. The area was not only a part of the original Stephen F. Austin land grant in the 1820s but also an earlier home to the Karankawa Indians, whose reported cannibalistic habits now only seem fitting, considering the park's most popular current resident, the American alligator. Throw in a specific warning for venomous snakes and you have a good chance to observe wild animals in their habitat.

As you leave US 59 and turn onto FM 762, you soon pass the outer limits of suburbia and the George Ranch Historical Park on your right. Follow FM 762 for 11.4 miles, then enter the park on Park Road 72. The headquarters is straight ahead and surrounded by massive live oaks covered with Spanish moss. On a clear, sunny day, you sense this camping and hiking experience will have some significant rewards. On a foggy, rainy day, you will feel as if the prehistoric world of dinosaurs awaits you.

At 0.3 mile, you'll spot a large picnic area on your left, overlooking the 40-acre lake. Be sure to check out the multiple nature programs offered at this popular park, such as photo walks, bird-watching events, and of course, the Gatorwise Club for those young tent campers looking to satisfy their curiosity about these prehistoric descendants. As you continue

Enjoy the peaceful view at Brazos Bend . . .

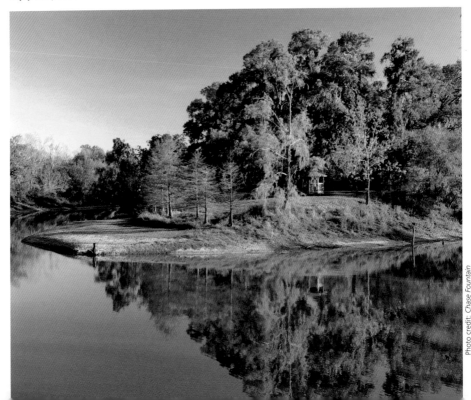

Photo credit: Chase Fountain

KEY INFORMATION

ADDRESS: 21901 FM 762,
Needville, TX 77461

CONTACT: 979-553-5101, brazosbend.org,
tpwd.texas.gov/state-parks/brazos-bend

OPERATED BY: Texas Parks & Wildlife
Department

OPEN: Year-round

SITES: 73; 8 walk-in; 13 shelters

EACH SITE: Picnic table, fire ring, water,
electricity, lantern hook

ASSIGNMENT: First come, first served
until site-specific reservation system
begins in 2018

REGISTRATION: At headquarters or reserve
at texas.reserveworld.com or
512-389-8900

FACILITIES: Restrooms with showers, walk-in
sites with water & restrooms nearby,
nature center, observatory, gift shop,
museum, youth group primitive camping area

PARKING: At each site

FEE: $12–$20; shelters $25; $7/person
entrance fee, age 12 and under free

ELEVATION: 74'

RESTRICTIONS:

PETS: On leash only

FIRES: In fire rings

ALCOHOL: Prohibited in all public/
outdoor areas

VEHICLES: 2/site

OTHER: Maximum 8 people/site; guests must
leave by 10 p.m.; quiet time 10 p.m.–
6 a.m.; bring your own firewood or charcoal; limited supplies at park headquarters
and gift store; pick up main supplies in
Richmond, Sugarland, or Houston

---

on the main road, the huge trees begin to close over the pavement to form a canopy of shade. You will begin to notice the lowlands on both sides of the road for 2.5 miles until you reach the large parking lot at the nature center, where hands-on exhibits attract the kids, and helpful volunteers suggest the best gator viewing areas.

Across the street are two must-see sites. The first is the George Observatory, with three domed telescopes and public viewings on Saturdays 3–10 p.m. Call 979-553-3400 for details. The other is the 0.5-mile Creekfield Interpretive Trail, which circles Creekfield Lake for some close-up views of the local waterfowl. With the park's proximity to the Texas coast and its status as part of the Brazos River floodplain, the chance to see more than 300 species makes this a birdwatcher's and photographer's gold mine.

Returning to the main road, turn right to the Burr Oak Camping Area and sites 100–141. These large sites have electricity and a fair number of RVs. Fortunately, they are spacious, with sites 120–123 and 106 and 107 located on the ends for a little extra privacy to spread out into the woods.

Leaving Burr Oak, stay to the right for the Red Buckeye Camping Area sites 200–234. This area also has electrified RVs, but sites 215–217 and 232–234 give the best chance for some solitude. Be sure to ask about the new walk-in tent-only area sites.

As you complete the Red Buckeye Circle, screened shelter sites 1–13 offer a good alternative to the RV areas. Pitch your tent outside the shelter and use it for a mosquito escape or severe storm shelter if necessary.

Returning to the main road, turn right toward Elm Lake and a chance to see some wetland areas that truly qualify as wild lands. Following the 1.7-mile Elm Lake Loop Trail, you immediately see large areas of disturbed mud and brush along the shoreline. It looks as if a truck or tractor went off the elevated pathway, but you soon learn these are the unmistakable signs of the American alligator. Of particular interest on the day I hiked was a very large 10- to 11-foot gator happily sunning himself on a small island just 40 or 50 feet from the hikers quickly snapping pictures and holding onto their small children. After seeing this massive animal enjoying a midday nap, you understand the necessity for "alligator etiquette" and keeping your dogs on a short leash away from the water.

While the alligators (and all the others) move throughout the park, you have 22 miles of hiking and mountain-bike trails to enjoy this premier destination just a little more than an hour from the Houston skyline and its own cement jungle. So when you need a break, come here for a taste of the real jungle. You won't be disappointed.

VOICES FROM THE CAMPFIRE AND RECOMMENDED READING

It is not enough to understand the natural world; the point is to defend and preserve it.
Edward Abbey, *A Voice Crying in the Wilderness* (New York, St. Martin's Press, 1989).

Writing, at its best, is a lonely life. . . . For he does his work alone, and if he is a good enough writer, he must face eternity, or the lack of it, each day.

For a true writer, each book should be a new beginning where he tries again for something that is beyond attainment. He should always try for something that has never been done or that others have tried and failed. Then sometimes, with great luck, he will succeed.

(Ernest Hemingway, "Banquet Speech" (Nobel Prize in Literature speech, Stockholm, Sweden, December 10, 1954), Nobel Prize, nobelprize.org/nobel_prizes/literature/laureates/1954/hemingway-speech.html.

. . . but do watch your gator etiquette!

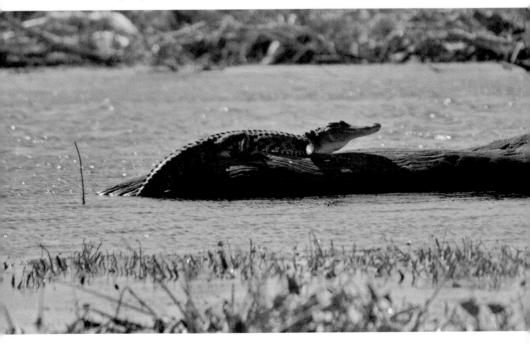

BACKCOUNTRY ADVENTURES

Even a casual stroll along the raised pathways of this park will get your heart beating a little quicker. Because the alligators, snakes, and all other wild animals are protected by law, they are on home territory; you are the visitor. Follow all the signage and directions from the park rangers so you don't end up in an accident report. As always, feeding any of the animals is strictly forbidden. I wonder about one parent who was letting his small boy throw rocks at a nice 10-foot alligator trying to get some sun on a winter day.

BEST LOCAL FOOD AND DRINK

While Houston can get you all the fast-food chains you want to avoid, in Needville try The Jay Café (979-793-7900) for a home-cooked breakfast, Los Charros (979-793-7799), or 36 Bar and Grill (979-793-4403) for a great burger.

Brazos Bend State Park

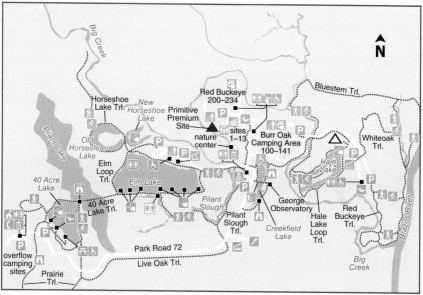

GETTING THERE

From the western intersection of I-69 and I-610 in Houston, drive southwest on I-69 for 17.5 miles. Take the exit toward FM 2759/Crabb River Road/Grand Pkwy. Turn left onto Crabb River Road and drive 2.4 miles. Continue onto FM 762 and drive 5 miles. Keep left to stay on FM 762 and drive another 3.3 miles. Again turn left to stay on FM 762 and drive 5.8 miles; the park entrance will be on your left.

GPS COORDINATES: N29° 22.248' W95° 37.884'

29

⛺ Choke Canyon State Park

Beauty: ★★★ / Privacy: ★★ / Spaciousness: ★★★ / Quiet: ★★★★ / Security: ★★★ / Cleanliness: ★★★

With names like Owl Hollow, Hawk Alley, and Dove Place, you know to bring your binoculars, spotting scopes, and long-range camera lenses.

As you travel through the heavy brush country of South Texas between Corpus Christi and San Antonio, the Choke Canyon Reservoir is a true oasis. This Bureau of Reclamation project not only provides a water supply for human visitors but also serves as a prime birding area. Throw in a few alligators and you have an ideal destination for tent campers.

Leaving the park's headquarters, you will notice deer-crossing signs, healthy cacti, mesquite grasslands, and widespread Tamaulipan thorn shrubs. Turn right at the T-intersection to head toward the camping areas and tent sites 200–215. The 75-acre lake is on the immediate right; sites 206–215 have clear views of this small lake and the numerous birds enjoying its protected shores. Don't be fooled, though, by its calmness; a quick look at the shore vegetation reveals a good deal of disturbance by the local alligators. The tent sites are elevated from the shoreline, but do follow the park instructions for "alligator etiquette."

Continue on the circle to sites 200–205 for premium waterfront sites on the main reservoir. You get all the benefits of the lake breeze here, plus sunrise views over a large portion of the lake without an RV in sight.

The freedom of flight

KEY INFORMATION

ADDRESS: County Road 302/Recreational Road 8, Calliham, TX 78007

CONTACT: 361-786-3868, tpwd.texas.gov/state-parks/choke-canyon

OPERATED BY: Texas Parks & Wildlife Department

OPEN: Year-round

SITES: 16 tent-only sites, 20 shelter sites

EACH SITE: Picnic table, fire ring, lantern hook

ASSIGNMENT: First come, first served until site-specific reservation system begins in 2018

REGISTRATION: At headquarters or reserve at texas.reserveworld.com or 512-389-8900

FACILITIES: Modern restrooms and showers, boat ramp, rock jetty, sponsored youth-group area

PARKING: Near each site

FEE: $12 walk-in waterfront sites; $5/person entrance fee, age 12 and under free

ELEVATION: 196'

RESTRICTIONS:

PETS: On leash only

FIRES: In fire rings with grates; check on burn bans

ALCOHOL: Prohibited in all public/outdoor areas

VEHICLES: 2/site

OTHER: Maximum 8 people/site; guests must leave by 10 p.m.; quiet time 10 p.m.– 6 a.m.; firewood sold at park or bring your own; bring charcoal; ice and groceries available in Three Rivers; pick up main supplies in San Antonio or Corpus Christi; gathering firewood prohibited

As you return to the main road, a number of bird-watching trails have been cleared from the dense vegetation. With names like Owl Hollow, Hawk Alley, and Dove Place, you know to bring your binoculars, spotting scopes, and long-range camera lenses. In addition to permanent residents, such as the long-billed and curve-billed thrashers, look for Audubon's orioles and brown-crested and vermillion flycatchers, along with nearly 300 other species listed in the field checklist available at the park headquarters.

Continuing on the main road, turn left into the shelter area for tent-camping sites 1–20. Look for sites 12–20 for great waterfront and sunset views. This area would be especially attractive if your group contains non–tent campers or the weather turns unexpectedly dangerous. Just reserve a shelter and put your tent up next door in the surrounding grassy area. You get the great water view, and the RVs are down the road and out of sight.

After locating your tent site, grab your hiking partner and head into the heavy bush. Birds are literally all around as you explore more than 12,500 acres in this wildlife management area. When you return to the picnic area, keep an eye out for cave swallows that nest under the roofs of shelters. While many of the bird species pass through at various times of the year, the park is most popular in winter when the warm South Texas weather attracts bird enthusiasts from all over the world. However, be aware that a sudden cold snap can arrive without much warning, so pack your heavy sleeping bag just in case. During late spring, summer, and early fall, the heat and humidity can be a real danger to day hikers who walk too far from their tent without sufficient water, a wide-brimmed hat, or sunscreen.

As you leave the park and turn left for 7.3 miles, be sure to visit the South Shore Unit and the area below the dam. This riparian woodland area is home to shorebirds, herons, egrets, and even passerines. It also follows the Frio River, which was dammed to create Choke Canyon Reservoir and provide abundant fishing opportunities in the 75-acre lake stocked with bass, bluegill, white crappie, and channel catfish.

VOICES FROM THE CAMPFIRE AND RECOMMENDED READING

We need wilderness because we are wild animals. Every man needs a place where he can go to go crazy in peace. Every Boy Scout troop deserves a forest to get lost, miserable, and starving in.
Edward Abbey, *The Journey Home: Some Words in Defense of the American West* (New York, Dutton, 1977).

This is a delicious evening, when the whole body is one sense, and imbibes delight through every pore. I go and come with a strange liberty in Nature, a part of herself. As I walk along the stony shore of the pond in my shirtsleeves, though it is cool as well as cloudy and windy, and I see nothing special to attract me, all the elements are unusually congenial to me. The bullfrogs trump to usher in the night, and the note of the whip-poor-will is borne on the rippling wind from over the water.
Henry David Thoreau, *Walden and Other Writings* (New York, Random House Inc., 1965). Solitude, Journal, 1840–1841

BACKCOUNTRY ADVENTURES

While birding or going on an easy canoe ride are not always in the adventure category, a fair number of local alligators does add some interest to who might answer your birdcalls. To the south, you can also stop in at Lake Corpus Christi State Park for additional tent-camping sites and one of the best CCC-built buildings known as the Refectory.

As ancient as dinosaurs and alligators, just a little smaller

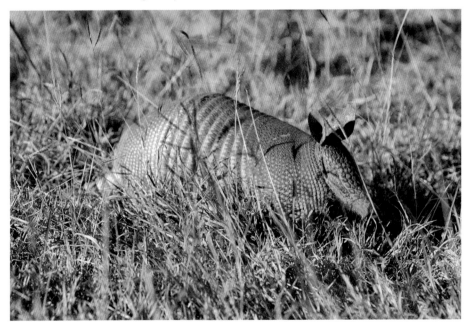

BEST LOCAL FOOD AND DRINK

In Three Rivers, try Sowell's BBQ (361-786-3333) on your way into the park, and the Staghorn (361-786-3545) or Agave Jalisco (361-786-4050; agavejalisco.com) on your way out. Try Taqueria Vallarta if going south, through Mathis (361-547-8041).

Choke Canyon State Park

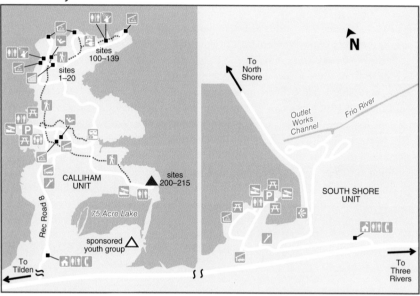

GETTING THERE

From I-37 exit onto TX 72 W and drive 11 miles. Follow the signs in Three Rivers and pass South Shore Day-Use Area. Turn right onto County Road 302/Recreational Road 8. Park headquarters is 1.3 miles ahead.

GPS COORDINATES: N28° 27.966' W98° 21.252'

30

Goose Island State Park

Beauty: ★★★★ / Privacy: ★★★ / Spaciousness: ★★★ / Quiet: ★★★ / Security: ★★★ / Cleanliness: ★★★

Three hundred recorded species, including the magnificent whooping crane, make this portion of the Texas coast a bird-watcher's gold mine.

Don't be fooled by the size of this 314-acre park. Goose Island State Park sits in the middle of some of the most important and beautiful natural areas of Texas. Whether you are coming from the northeast through miles and miles of the 59,000-acre Aransas National Wildlife Refuge or from the southwest and the white beaches of Corpus Christi, always be alert for some incredible wildlife. Even an old abandoned farmstead on TX 35 can provide the view of a lifetime. I spotted a pair of whooping cranes (a critically endangered species) near sunset here, less than 75 yards from the roadside during the peak winter bird-watching season. These magnificent five-foot-tall birds—along with 300 other recorded species—make this portion of the Texas coast a bird-watcher's gold mine.

For the tent camper, an immediate right after the entrance station into the wooded area brings you to sites 201–203. This area of dense trees provides a welcome bit of shade in this expanse of open coastal vegetation. Continuing on the Lantana Loop, tent sites 207–209 are close to the road, with sites 210–218 back in the woods for extra privacy. If these sites are full, consider sites 151 and 152, which have electricity but are divided by heavy-enough brush to shield your tent from any nearby RVs. When you pass site 157, also look for the 0.66-mile Turks Cap Trail for a close-up view of local bird life.

This coastal live oak and the Texas coast have survived a few hurricanes.

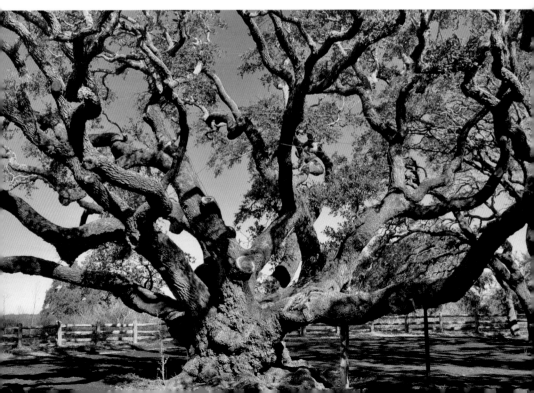

KEY INFORMATION

ADDRESS: 202 S. Palmetto St., Rockport, TX 78382

CONTACT: 361-729-2858, tpwd.texas.gov/state-parks/goose-island

OPERATED BY: Texas Parks & Wildlife Department

OPEN: Year-round

SITES: 125

EACH SITE: Picnic table, fire rings/grates, central water, lantern hooks

ASSIGNMENT: First come, first served until site-specific reservation system begins in 2018

REGISTRATION: At headquarters or reserve at texas.reserveworld.com or 512-389-8900

FACILITIES: Boat ramp, fishing pier, restrooms with showers

PARKING: Near each site

FEE: $10 (basic); $5/person entrance fee, age 12 and under free

ELEVATION: 26' below sea level

RESTRICTIONS:

PETS: On leash only

FIRES: In fire rings

ALCOHOL: Prohibited in all public/ outdoor areas

VEHICLES: 2/site

OTHER: Maximum 8 people/site; guests must leave by 10 p.m.; quiet time 10 p.m.– 6 a.m.; bring your own firewood or charcoal; limited supplies at park store; pick up main supplies in Rockport or Corpus Christi; gathering firewood prohibited. *Note:* This area was especially hard hit by Hurricane Harvey in August 2017. Call ahead or check the park website for specific recovery updates.

Once you set up camp, the real adventure begins. Serious birdwatchers, photographers, and fishermen should return to the main road and turn right toward the Bay Front Area and the Recreation Hall Area, with its tall palm trees and resort feel. This is the meeting point for many of the guided nature tours that may come upon some of the whooping cranes that reside in the park and surrounding wetlands. There are also ample fishing opportunities for speckled trout, redfish, drum, flounder, and sheepshead. Photographers should follow the road across the small bridge for Bayfront sites 1–44. While these sites attract RVs, the sunset view across the bay toward Corpus Christi is perfect for that low-light exposure. Be sure you have a tripod if the herons agree to pose in a perfect spot just off the bank.

Returning to park headquarters, travel straight on Park Road 13 north toward the Big Tree. This state champion coastal live oak is estimated to be more than 1,000 years old, with a circumference of 35 feet and a crown of 90 feet. It is also close to Fourth Street Pond, where the black-crowned night herons roost, joined by an occasional yellow-crowned night heron and especially abundant warblers. Whatever your reason for visiting, put down your tent and stay a few days in this wildlife bonanza.

VOICES FROM THE CAMPFIRE AND RECOMMENDED READING

The sight of a Whooping Crane in the air is an experience packed with beauty and drama. We see the broad sweep of the great wings in their stiff, almost ponderous motion, the flash of sunlight on the satin white plumage.

Robert Porter Allen, *The Whooping Crane* (New York, National Audubon Society, 1952).

I also recommend *Return of the Whooping Crane* by Robin W. Doughty (University of Texas Press, 1989).

BACKCOUNTRY ADVENTURES

This part of Texas coast has two premier adventures. The first is the whooping crane tour boat, which leaves from Rockport (Rockport Adventures: 877-892-4737; rockportadventures .com). Captain Tommy has an incredible eye for the "whoopers" and the thousands of other birds in the hidden coves and wetlands.

The second adventure is the Aransas National Wildlife Refuge about an hour to the northeast from Rockport. Plan on a half day here to experience this true piece of wilderness. The refuge has various tours to make sure you get the full experience. The refuge has the largest number of whooping cranes in North America. A 16-mile auto tour features numerous exhibits and viewing areas. The alligator viewing area is a treat for the whole family. Don't miss it.

BEST LOCAL FOOD AND DRINK

The nearby city of Rockport has enough restaurants for all you hungry tent campers. Start at Alby's (361-729-1521; albysseafood.com) on TX 35 for the best catfish po'boys around. Finish the day at Charlotte Plummer's Seafare Restaurant (361-729-1185; charlotteplummers .com) and try the crab tower, or go to the Boiling Pot (361-729-6972) for Cajun seafood.

Note: Rockport took a direct hit from Hurricane Harvey in 2017, so inquire ahead of time to see which restaurants have reopened.

Goose Island State Park

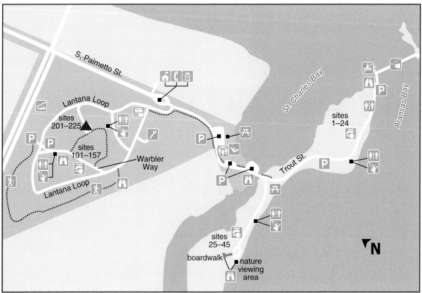

GETTING THERE

From Rockport, travel 12 miles northeast on TX 35. Turn right onto Main St./Park Road 13 and drive 1.4 miles. Turn right onto S. Palmetto St./Park Road 13B and drive to the park entrance.

GPS COORDINATES: N28° 7.986' W96° 59.052'

31

Mustang Island State Park

Beauty: ★★★★ / Privacy: ★★★ / Spaciousness: ★★★★ / Quiet: ★★★★ / Security: ★★★ / Cleanliness: ★★★

The simple act of walking for miles on the white-sand beaches will bring you back every year.

Named after the herds of wild mustangs that roamed this area until the late 1800s, this premier tent-camping area is located on the beach, only 20 miles from downtown Corpus Christi. As you approach the sand dunes, the RV sites are to the left in a parking lot where you cannot see the beach or the ocean but where you'll find showers and restrooms. Continuing on, turn right toward Beach Camping and the crashing waves become your constant companion, along with seagulls overhead. Using the beach as your roadway, look for a prime spot to pitch your tent. The 50 newly marked tent-camping sites dictate where you can set up camp, but you will still enjoy plenty of space between your neighbors. Remember that the dunes are part of a fragile ecosystem and they are the only real protection for the island, so don't stray off the beach. There are also snakes in the dunes in case you need another reason to stay off.

After securely staking down your tent and putting on the rainfly in case of a squall line off the gulf, begin winding down from whatever stress you had in the city. There are more than 400 bird species that either live on the island or pass through during migratory season, so a pair of binoculars or a good telephoto lens will add to your experience. You might also enjoy some extended beachcombing. Periodic storms and crashing waves constantly bring in new seashells, along with food for a wide range of shorebirds, including the quick plovers, killdeers, and sandpipers darting beside the stately herons, long-billed curlews, and ponderous pelicans. The fishing is also excellent from the jetty or the shore, but the real enjoyment here lies in the therapeutic waves and the almost-constant sea breeze. When you add the unlimited views

A walk on the beach with the family

KEY INFORMATION

ADDRESS: 17047 TX 361, Port Aransas, TX 78373

CONTACT: 361-749-5246, tpwd.texas.gov/state-parks/mustang-island

OPERATED BY: Texas Parks & Wildlife Department

OPEN: Year-round

SITES: 50 on the beach, 48 RV/tent sites

EACH SITE: Central water, portable toilets, rinsing showers nearby

ASSIGNMENT: First come, first served until site-specific reservation system begins in 2018

REGISTRATION: At entrance station or reserve at texas.reserveworld.com or 512-389-8900

FACILITIES: Modern restrooms and showers

PARKING: At each site

FEE: $10 beach camping; $5/person entrance fee, age 12 and under free

ELEVATION: 6'

RESTRICTIONS:

PETS: On leash only

FIRES: In fire rings only

ALCOHOL: Prohibited in all public/outdoor areas

VEHICLES: 2/site

OTHER: Maximum 8 people/site; guests must leave by 10 p.m.; quiet time 10 p.m.–6 a.m.; bring your own firewood or charcoal; limited supplies at park store; pick up main supplies in Corpus Christi; gathering firewood prohibited. *Note:* This park took a hit from Hurricane Harvey, which devastated Rockport, in August 2017. Call to check on current conditions.

to the horizon, the simple act of walking for miles on the white-sand beaches will bring you back every year, even if that lightning-fast seagull stole your lunch when you weren't looking.

Large storms often wash up some extra debris, so remember to pack up your trash so the seabirds don't mistake it for food. There can also be a strong undertow not too far off the shoreline, along with a stinging jellyfish or two. Whatever your activity, a little extra caution will make this seaside beauty a tent camper's real paradise. Extreme wet and muddy conditions can cause problems at certain entrances, so call the park office ahead of time to hear "closed area information" on their message options.

Heading inland, notice the intricate set of dunes that also protects the island from the occasional hurricane. These deep-rooted coastal grasses and vines are essential to preventing beach erosion from both wind and storm surges. They also protect the area's small mammals, such as pocket gophers, ground squirrels, mice, and cotton rats. These important inhabitants are key food sources for the soaring hawks as well as coyotes and bobcats. While these animals may be hard to find during the day, their tracks will be a reminder that barrier islands are an ecosystem worth protecting.

VOICES FROM THE CAMPFIRE AND RECOMMENDED READING

On a warm, windy day in March, I watched as a great blue heron paced the shallows along the Rockport waterfront, leaning into the brisk sea breeze for balance. Turning its head to focus one eye on the choppy water just ahead, it slowed its pace to a careful stalk. Then, in a motion almost too fast to follow, it drove its head beneath the surface, emerging with a foot-long mullet impaled on its rapier beak. . . . Looking around as if for approval, the heron then fluffed its long neck plumes in the wind, walked a few strides into the surf, and launched into ponderous flight.
John L. Tveten, *The Birds of Texas* (Fredericksburg, TX, Shearer Publishing, 1993).

BACKCOUNTRY ADVENTURES

On a gray, windy, winter day you would expect to see only a few beach walkers. However, on Mustang Island you may be joined by the stunning skill and fearlessness of the kite surfers racing along the shoreline. Their ability to move far out into the rough surf and then return to the shore area with apparent ease will leave you breathless. This was not a day for beginners, but the intrepid camper might be inspired to give it a try with professional instruction.

BEST LOCAL FOOD AND DRINK

Near the intersection of TX 361 and JFK Causeway is the very authentic JB's German Bakery & Cafe (361-949-5474; jbsgermanbakery.com). The owners are German natives who came to the Texas coast and decided to stay. The menu is extensive and will transport all your senses to a small German village. The next stop is a little Texan—check out Padre Island Burger Company (361-949-3490; padreislandburgercompany.com). Scuttlebutts Seafood Bar & Grill (361-949-6769; scuttlebuttsbarandgrill.com) is also a favorite of the locals.

Mustang Island State Park

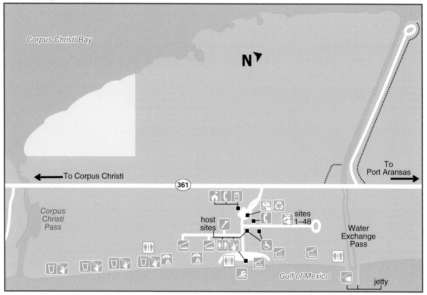

GETTING THERE

From Corpus Christi, cross the JFK Causeway. Turn left onto TX 361 N and drive about 5 miles. The park entrance will be on your right.

GPS COORDINATES: N27° 40.332' W97° 10.464'

32

⚠ Padre Island National Seashore

Beauty: ★★★★ / Privacy: ★★★ / Spaciousness: ★★★★★ (on the beach) / Quiet: ★★★★ (on the beach) / Security: ★★★ / Cleanliness: ★★★★

A few days at Padre Island National Seashore will help shake whatever big-city ills you brought along.

As you leave the city of Corpus Christi, the wide-open spaces of the world's longest undeveloped stretch of barrier island beckons you like a siren's song. For those tent campers who live too far inland, a yearly journey to Padre Island National Seashore is an essential requirement for renewing the soul in a way that only a great body of untamed water can. As you look over the waves to an endless horizon, you instantly begin to feel the big city leave you, and a primal connection to the earth returns.

Approaching the park entrance on Park Road 22, miles and miles of grass-covered sand dunes flank the way. There are no buildings in sight, and even the old cattle fences have been removed. Depending on the latest storm, the roadway may still have blown sand along the way, which only adds to the anticipation. Prior to the entrance station, the North Beach Access Road to your left allows camping and is also a popular day-use area. Passing into the national seashore, you'll see a nature trail at 0.2 mile on your right and the Bird Island Basin turnoff in 0.7 mile. Continue on for 2.5 miles and turn left onto 20410 Park Road, heading for the Malaquite Beach Campground. This is primarily an RV campground, but there are six tent-only sites, along with restrooms and showers. The beach is somewhat hidden by the dunes, but the picnic tables on the beach are closer to the water.

Easy bayside camping

KEY INFORMATION

ADDRESS: 20420 Park Road 22, Corpus Christi, TX 78418

CONTACT: 361-949-8068 or 361-949-8173, nps.gov/pais; no reservations accepted

OPERATED BY: National Park Service

OPEN: Year-round

SITES: 6 tent sites in Malaquite, 6 unmarked sites at Bird Island Basin, unlimited sites on beach.

EACH SITE: Malaquite has a picnic table with a shelter; Bird Island Basin has a picnic table with a shelter and a grill

ASSIGNMENT: First come, first served

REGISTRATION: At visitor center or self-registration kiosks

FACILITIES: Visitor center, park store, restrooms with cold showers, potable water

PARKING: At each site

FEE: $8 (Malaquite); $5 (Bird Island Basin); no charge (beach); $10/vehicle entrance fee

ELEVATION: 11'

RESTRICTIONS:

PETS: On leash only

FIRES: In fire rings

ALCOHOL: Prohibited

VEHICLES: 2/site

OTHER: Maximum 8 people/site; guests must leave by 10 p.m.; quiet time 10 p.m.–6 a.m.; bring your own firewood or charcoal; limited supplies at visitor center

Leaving Malaquite, the visitor center is only 1 mile away, but the change in feeling is distinct. While the parking lot is large, the center itself is built into the landscape with classic "parkitecture," such that you have a sense of approaching a frontier outpost, not a government building. The rustic decking and skin-saving shade structures house the small museum, a park store, and modern restrooms with excellent showers. There are also elevated platforms for not only ocean views but also your first look far down the beach and sand dunes where you see . . . more beach and sand dunes. Even from the visitor center, you begin to realize this is the start of a very large stretch of wilderness where everyone can spread out and have the type of space modern society so often lacks.

As you leave the parking lot, the paved road curves between the sand dunes, and the white sands become your new highway. The self-registration station is on your immediate right, where you pick up your free backcountry use permit. Proceeding on the beach, which is considered a public highway in Texas, you drive on the firm sand near the crashing waves, but not too near. In choosing a site, you have the first 5 miles to pick the amount of space desired between you and any other campers. There are periodic portable toilets, which may also impact your choice.

If you have a four-wheel drive, you can extend your wilderness camping range another 60 miles or so, but keep in mind the sand is very unpredictable, and even a four-wheel drive may get stuck. Regardless of where you choose to set up camp, a tent pad in the soft sand is a true outdoor luxury. Add the constant sound of the waves, the calling seabirds, and the cooling breeze, and you have a premier tent-camping experience. Just be sure to stake down your tent and put on your rainfly, because those beautiful towering clouds way out on the Gulf might come your way in the middle of the night. If they do, it will still be a great camping experience to hold your tent walls with both arms outstretched and then tell all your friends how you survived the raging storm from the high seas while your fellow car camper jumped in the backseat of the vehicle.

Returning to the visitor center for a necessary shower, keep a close watch for the often-hidden Kemp's Ridley sea turtle nests or even the highly endangered turtles themselves, or their offspring "racing" for the water and freedom. From June to August, Padre Island National Seashore is home to these amazing creatures, whose popularity has caused more than 3,000 people to attend releases of the incubated hatchlings back to the sea.

Head back toward the front-entrance gate, and the turnoff for Bird Island Basin is on your left. This campground and day-use area is the new hot spot in the park, where wind-surfing on the usually placid Laguna Madre attracts surfers from all over the country. Rentals and lessons are available, along with tent camping at the far end of the RV/camper sites. The tent sites are unnumbered, but six parking spots have been set aside for tent campers.

Whether you are racing across the Laguna Madre or walking on the beach alongside sea birds racing the tides, spending a few days at Padre Island National Seashore will help shake whatever big-city ills you showed up with.

VOICES FROM THE CAMPFIRE AND RECOMMENDED READING

A wild place without dangers is an absurdity, although I realize that danger creates administrative problems for park and forest managers. But we must not allow our national parks and national forests to be degraded to the status of mere public playgrounds. Open to all, yes of course. But—enter at your own risk.

Edward Abbey, *The Journey Home: Some Words in Defense of the American West* (New York, Dutton, 1977).

Because all organisms have descended from a common ancestor, it is correct to say that the biosphere as a whole began to think when humanity was born. If the rest of life is the body, we are the mind. Thus, our place in nature, viewed from an ethical perspective, is to think about the creation and to protect the living planet.

Edward O. Wilson, *The Future of Life* (New York, Alfred A. Knopf, 2002).

Even a little shade helps.

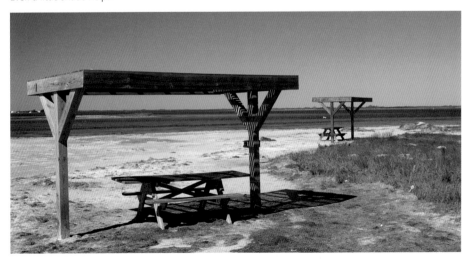

BACKCOUNTRY ADVENTURES

The Bird Island Basin is a great place to observe and even learn windsurfing. Lessons and rentals that will get you started are available on-site. Just remember that while the Laguna Madre can be like a glass lake, the proximity of the ocean just a few hundred yards over the dunes can bring out Texas-force winds, leaving you trying to hang on to your gear.

BEST LOCAL FOOD AND DRINK

Just after you cross the JFK Causeway, coming from Corpus Christi, take an immediate right toward two of the best seafood restaurants along the Texas coast: Doc's Seafood & Steaks (361-949-6744; docsseafoodandsteaks.com) and Snoopy's Pier (361-949-8815; snoopyspier .com). There, bayside dining places serve fish as fresh as you can catch it, and even the most basic fare tastes better than those fancy places in the big cities from which you are escaping. Look for their daily specials to get the best of the best. After a very filling meal, you are really ready for the wilderness experience ahead of you.

Padre Island National Seashore

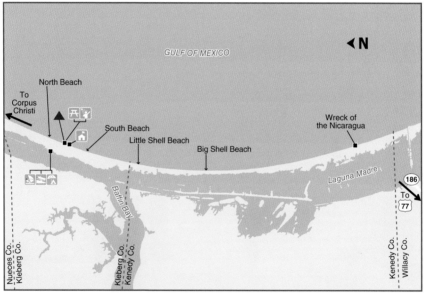

GETTING THERE

From the intersection of US 286 and US 358 in Corpus Christi, take TX 358 E and drive 9.4 miles. Continue onto John F. Kennedy Memorial Causeway (signs for Park Road 22/ Padre Island) and drive 5 miles. Continue onto S. Padre Island Dr./PR 22 and drive 10.6 miles to the park entrance.

GPS COORDINATES: N27° 25.482' W97° 17.916'

33

⚕ Texana Park and Campground

Beauty: ★★★ / Privacy: ★★★ / Spaciousness: ★★★ / Quiet: ★★★★ / Security: ★★★★ / Cleanliness: ★★★★

Hiking trails leading from the Texana trailhead are perfect for wildlife photography and solitude.

Located between Houston and Victoria off US 59, this campground seems remote to human travelers, but is situated perfectly for migratory birds heading to and from the Texas coast. As you enter the park, heavy tree cover protects you. Once you take an immediate left across the bridge, wildlife appears near the road, including the armor-plated armadillo and the majestic great blue heron searching for food in a backwater cove starved for rain during years of drought. You also see the Texana trailhead, which connects to approximately 4.5 miles of hiking trails that are perfect for wildlife photography and solitude. Although this park is no longer part of the Texas State Park system, it still has much to offer. The water-only sites are gone, but tent camping is allowed in any of the partial, full, and pull-through sites, except for the camping circles located in Brackenridge Park.

Continuing straight on the main road, you'll see sites 1–26, arranged on both sides of the road for easy access. After site 26, make a hard right for much-larger sites 27 and 29, which back up to the cove for premier waterfront views. Continue on to site 31 for not only water views but also an end location shaded by a huge tree. While all 14 lakeside sites are very good, choose 39 and 42 for easiest access to the lighted fishing pier; move farther away for privacy and darkness. The interior sites are also well spaced, with heavy brush shielding many of them from the neighboring tents.

Returning to the main road, continue across the second bridge into the area with multiple sites on the main Lake Texana. Turn right toward the nature center for canoe and kayak

This is a good park for families and novice campers.

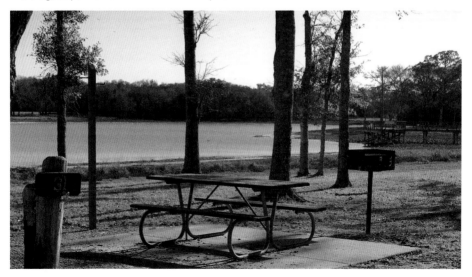

KEY INFORMATION

ADDRESS: 46 Park Road 1, Edna, TX 77957

CONTACT: 361-782-5718,
brackenridgepark.com (reservations)

OPERATED BY: Lavaca-Navidad
River Authority

OPEN: Year-round

SITES: 141

EACH SITE: Picnic table, fire ring and grate,
lantern hook, central water

ASSIGNMENT: Specific sites can be chosen
when making reservations online

REGISTRATION: At park entrance

FACILITIES: Modern restrooms and showers,
lighted fishing pier, park store

PARKING: At each site

FEE: $25–$30/night; no entrance fee for
campers

ELEVATION: 20'

RESTRICTIONS:

PETS: On leash only

FIRES: In fire rings

ALCOHOL: Prohibited

VEHICLES: 2/site

OTHER: Maximum 8 people/site; quiet time
11 p.m.–10 a.m.; bring your own firewood
or charcoal; pick up main supplies in Edna,
Victoria, or Ganado; gathering firewood
prohibited

rentals. These normally peaceful modes of transportation may come with a little extra adventure, given the presence of a few American alligators basking under the watchful gaze of red-headed turkey vultures. These massive but elegant and sleek birds sit in dead trees observing the tourists picnicking on the water's edge. The birds patiently wait for the humans to depart, then swoop silently down for an evening meal of any food carelessly left behind.

Returning to your campsite, be sure to get to bed early. Sunrises over the lake are the perfect backdrop for photographing the white-tailed deer and the abundant bird life preparing to head back north as spring approaches. These birds include more than 225 species spending part of their winter in the park and the Matagorda Bay area just to the south. The birds then migrate along a narrow bottleneck on the great Central Flyway, which links North America with Central and South America. Depending on the time of year, look for shorebirds, waterfowl, gulls, terns, raptors, passerines, and maybe even a flock of Baird's sandpipers on their nonstop flight to or from the high Arctic.

While watching the birds, you can also fish for largemouth bass, crappie, and catfish along the 125 miles of shoreline. Of course, don't be too distracted to notice the signs of an American alligator. If you see disturbed mud and crushed shoreline brush that looks like a vehicle got stuck in it, just move to another spot, and continue enjoying your stay at this lesser-known but very interesting park.

VOICES FROM THE CAMPFIRE AND RECOMMENDED READING

Most men, even in this comparatively free country, through mere ignorance and mistake, are so occupied with the factitious cares and superfluously coarse labors of life that its finer fruits cannot be plucked by them.

. . . Most of the luxuries, and many of the so-called comforts of life, are not only not indispensable, but positive hindrances to the elevation of mankind.

Henry David Thoreau, *Walden* (Boston, Ticknor and Fields, 1854).

BACKCOUNTRY ADVENTURES

While this inland park seems a little far from the coast, it is actually located just a short drive from the Great Texas Coastal Birding Trail, which follows the general coastline of Texas and allows side-trip access to a number of hidden but very special places, such as Brazoria National Wildlife Refuge, San Bernard National Wildlife Refuge, and Big Boggy National Wildlife Refuge. These remote retreats have very limited services and hours open to the public. Local inquiry should be made as to road conditions and necessary gear. They can also have a healthy mosquito population in warmer months, so a winter visit is best.

BEST LOCAL FOOD AND DRINK

The nearby town of Edna offers the Pinto Bean Restaurant (361-781-0190) for good Mexican food. Edna's Seafood (361-782-9272) is also a favorite with the local crowd.

Texana Park and Campground

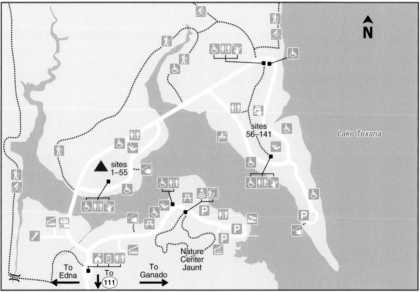

GETTING THERE

From the intersection of I-69 and I-610 in Houston, drive southwest on I-69 for 28.9 miles. Continue onto US 59 S and drive 54.6 miles. Take the exit for TX 172/TX 710/Ganado. Turn left onto FM 710, which quickly becomes N. Third St., and drive about 1.4 miles. Continue onto TX 172 S and drive 5.8 miles. Turn right onto TX 111 W and drive 3.9 miles. The park entrance will be on your right.

GPS COORDINATES: N28° 57.282' W96° 32.802'

THE TEXAS PANHANDLE, HIGH PLAINS, AND CAPROCK CANYONS

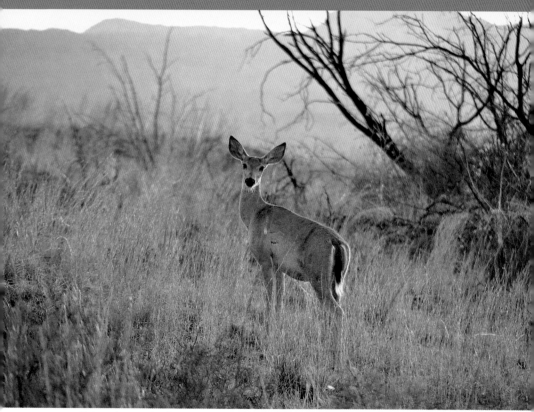

At sunset or sunrise, keep your camera ready. (Caprock Canyons State Park; see page 130)

34

⛺ Caprock Canyons State Park & Trailway

Beauty: ★★★★ / Privacy: ★★★ / Spaciousness: ★★★ / Quiet: ★★★★ / Security: ★★★★ / Cleanliness: ★★★★

Caprock Canyons State Park will immediately remind you of northern Arizona or southern Utah.

The high plains of Texas are an unlikely location for this hidden gem of a tent campground. However, a little perseverance and a short two-hour drive from either Lubbock or Amarillo will place you in a geological and historical setting that will immediately remind you of northern Arizona or southern Utah, complete with stunning red-rock formations, bison herds, and tales of Sioux, Crow, and Blackfoot tribes.

As you travel across the Panhandle, covering miles of tabletop-flat cotton fields, the sudden change of encountering the Caprock escarpment with its rugged hills and valleys is a welcome sight. The small town of Quitaque (pronounced "kitty-kway") is renovating its old main street buildings with the hope that visitors to this state park and its unique trail system will bring to the area a necessary revival.

Snow in the canyon country is always a treat; photo credit: *Chase Fountain*

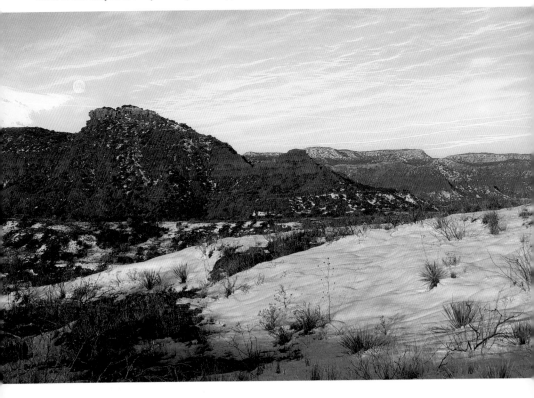

KEY INFORMATION

ADDRESS: 850 Caprock Canyon Park Road, Quitaque, TX 79255

CONTACT: 806-455-1492, tpwd.texas.gov /state-parks/caprock-canyons

OPERATED BY: Texas Parks & Wildlife Department

OPEN: Year-round

SITES: 49

EACH SITE: Amenities vary

ASSIGNMENT: First come, first served until site-specific reservation system begins in 2018

REGISTRATION: At entrance station or reserve at texas.reserveworld.com or 512-389-8900

FACILITIES: Restrooms and showers at RV area; restroom at Lake Theo; compost toilets at South Prong and Little Red areas

PARKING: Central parking

FEE: $14 (Lake Theo, Little Red walk-in); $12 (South Prong walk-in); $4/person entrance fee ($2/person with group, by prior arrangement)

ELEVATION: 2,569'

RESTRICTIONS:

PETS: On leash only

FIRES: Charcoal only in fire pits and grills; call ahead to check on fire danger level

ALCOHOL: Prohibited in all public/ outdoor areas

OTHER: Maximum 8 people/site; guests must leave by 10 p.m.; quiet time 10 p.m.– 6 a.m.; bring your own charcoal; no supplies at entrance station; limited supplies in Quitaque or Turkey

Leaving the main road (TX 86) and traveling north on FM 1065 for 3.5 miles, you will arrive at the visitor center to pay your fees and enjoy a fine overlook of Texas bison. Mary Ann and Charles Goodnight, who recognized that the bison were quickly becoming extinct, preserved a herd of native bison in the late 1870s on the famous JA Ranch, which is now Caprock Canyons. By 1929 the herd increased in number to around 250 and was used to help repopulate Yellowstone National Park. The herd now runs freely through a large section of the park and is a powerful symbol of this region of Texas and of how American Indians lived in harmony with the land before their conflict with Western expansion led to decades of war, relocation, and the near extermination of the bison.

Proceeding past the visitor center 0.5 mile, you arrive at Lake Theo and tent-camping sites 1–10. Look for the small gravel parking lot and a nice wide trail of about 100 yards that leads to the lakeside sites. Site 1 on the far left is on an elevated peninsula, which will provide a little extra airflow in the summer. The other sites are adequate, but the surrounding ground is not very level for pitching a tent. Unless you must have waterfront property, the other campsites will probably interest you more.

In the next 0.3 mile, the Honea Flat Campground turnoff leads you and the RV crowd to their allotted spaces and the only shower facilities in the park. These showers are more than adequate and this campground effectively keeps the larger vehicles away from the wilder areas of the park. Returning to the main park road, you begin to see the scale of red-rock beauty in this little-known park. This view of the canyon escarpment resembles a smaller version of the Vermillion Cliffs near the North Rim of the Grand Canyon and leads to the unique Wildhorse Campground, which allows you to bring horses along with your RV or trailer. While it's not a tent-camping area, the presence of horses and designated horse trails here echoes 19th-century cattle drives and the true Texas heritage of a cowboy surviving on the range many miles from home.

As you leave Wildhorse, the road drops at a 16% grade and begins a journey into the park, which will reward tent campers for their efforts. In 1.6 miles, turn into Little Red Tent Camping Area and park in the central parking lot. Tent sites 56–65 surround the lot and can be reached easily. Each site has a flat tent area, along with a covered picnic table, fire pit, and grill. The rustic composting toilets next to site 61 are clean and more than adequate. The sites all have excellent views over the canyon area, with site 65 perched perfectly overlooking the Little Red River. When staying at this small campsite, you forget the RVs and asphalt you left behind. As sunset approaches, you enjoy the sound of wind through the canyons and the pace of life slows to meet your own desires.

The final two stops are the North Prong Primitive Camping Area and the South Prong Tent Camping Area. The first requires a 1-mile backpacking hike, and the second contains tent sites 36–55, which have no covered tables and fire pits only. While these sites lack the seclusion of Little Red, they all share a 360-degree view of the red-rock formations and are close to the Upper Canyon Trail.

As in all areas of the park, be sure to remember you are in West Texas; while the local deer are cute and the bison magnificent, other wildlife includes rattlesnakes, which may not take kindly to you wandering off the trail.

As a final part of your visit, be sure to check out the Caprock Canyons Trailway, which crisscrosses the area for an incredible 64 miles. This trail system was created from abandoned railroad right-of-ways and features a 742-foot tunnel, complete with a resident population of Mexican free-tailed bats. The trail opened in 1993 as part of the Rails-to-Trails Conservancy program. It's the perfect addition to your stay.

VOICES FROM THE CAMPFIRE AND RECOMMENDED READING

A great deal of apprehension and misunderstanding still exist among Texans about their native serpents. In the minds of most persons, snakes are still the enemy. They are seen as mysterious and menacing, to be killed wherever and whenever they are encountered. The truth is that snakes—even the dangerous ones—are fundamentally shy and retiring, more than willing to avoid a confrontation with humans by fleeing when given the chance. Only as a last resort will they bite in self-defense.

James R. Dixon and John E. Werler, *Texas Snakes* (Austin, University of Texas Press, 2005).

BACKCOUNTRY ADVENTURES

Nothing provides excitement better than a leisurely morning hike that brings you within a few feet of a 1,200-pound bison and an equally large friend munching some wild grass by the trailside. While these two were luckily not interested in our little group of day hikers and we passed by quickly and quietly, the park now allows the entire herd to go where nature directs them, regardless of where tourists might stumble upon them. Since these bison and their ancestors have been there a few thousand years longer than we have, it is their home and our duty to allow them peace and space to enjoy the land. They will share, but on their terms. Just like the bison in Yellowstone National Park, these magnificent animals are wild and unpredictable. Give them plenty of space and the respect they deserve. Selfies are not recommended.

The other backcountry adventure not to be missed is the Caprock Canyon Trailway. At the park, you will encounter a number of cross-country bikers who use the facilities as their home base, adding some serious elevation changes and physical challenge to their trek.

BEST LOCAL FOOD AND DRINK

While there are a number of family-owned restaurants on US 287, you can wait for JB's Bar-B-Q (806-423-1512) in Turkey (open Wednesday–Saturday) or Dad's Barbeque (806-983-0619; d-bbq.com) in Quitaque near the park entrance. Be sure to call ahead because these and other small eateries in the area have limited days and hours of operation, but they are worth the stop. A "top-notch" stop in Childress is Top Notch Texas BBQ (940-937-8658; topnotchtexasbbq.com) on US 287. If you're looking for American food, visit Caprock Cafe (806-455-1429; caprockcafequitaque.com) in Quitaque. For a good meal and historical railroad ambience, get a table in the dining room at Hotel Turkey (806-423-1151; hotelturkeytexas.com).

Caprock Canyons State Park & Trailway

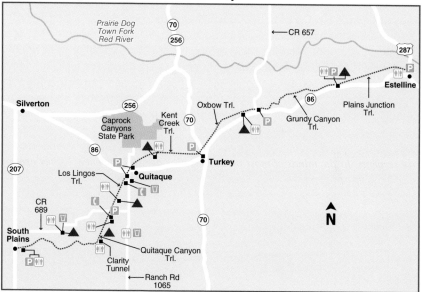

GETTING THERE

From the intersection of I-40 and I-27 in Amarillo, take I-27 S for 45.7 miles. Take Exit 77 for US 87/Tulia. Turn left onto US 87 S and drive 3.1 miles. Turn left onto TX 86 E and drive 44.5 miles. Turn left onto Ranch Road 1065 and drive 3 miles. Keep left where the road splits, and the park entrance will be straight ahead.

GPS COORDINATES: N34° 24.600' W101° 3.240'

35

Copper Breaks State Park

Beauty: ★★★★ / Privacy: ★★★ / Spaciousness: ★★★★ / Quiet: ★★★★ / Security: ★★★★ / Cleanliness: ★★★★

On a quiet day, you can easily imagine an early cowboy tending his campfire.

One of Texas's hidden gems, Copper Breaks State Park is a must-stop for tent campers, hikers, and history buffs. Don't be fooled by the approach from Quanah to the north or Crowell to the south. In an area where agriculture is practiced on such a large scale that the local crop duster has a fleet of planes, the Pease River and its tributaries have carved a "break" in the copper-rich hills for a rugged wilderness landscape sure to invite exploration.

As you enter the park, note the Texas longhorn herd on your left and prepare for a real history lesson about the early inhabitants of Texas. At the park's headquarters, there is a small but exceptional museum telling the story of fierce Comanches who hunted buffalo and protected their land against pioneers for more than 150 years. There is also the story of the legendary Quanah Parker, the last chief of the Staked Plains Comanches, whose Anglo mother was taken as a 9-year-old girl. She eventually married Chief Nocona, and when "found," she did not want to leave her Comanche family.

As you leave the headquarters and museum, note the warning about being in rattlesnake country and head into the park. As you travel the steep downhill grade of the road, the landscape instantly transforms from a flat prairie to multicolored rock cliffs lining the road; at the bottom, the trees begin to tower overhead. Take an immediate left into Kiowa Camping Area with 15 "civilized" tent sites near the modern restrooms and showers. The surrounding rocky hillsides and trees shelter this well-maintained area. The center area is

These West Texas campsites with a water view should not be missed.

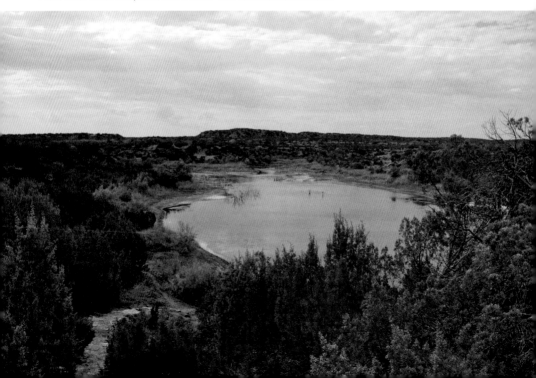

KEY INFORMATION

ADDRESS: 777 State Highway Park Road 62, Quanah, TX 79252

CONTACT: 817-839-4331, tpwd.texas.gov /state-parks/copper-breaks

OPERATED BY: Texas Parks & Wildlife Department

OPEN: Year-round

SITES: 11 in Kiowa, 10 in Big Pond; large tent site area available as 1 group or 4–5 individual sites in Big Pond and new Cottonwood areas

EACH SITE: Picnic table, fire ring, upright grill, lantern hook, water

ASSIGNMENT: First come, first served until site-specific reservation system begins in 2018

REGISTRATION: At headquarters or reserve at texas.reserveworld.com or 512-389-8900

FACILITIES: Modern restrooms at both areas, showers at Kiowa

PARKING: At each site

FEE: $10; $40 for group site; $2/person entrance fee, age 12 and under free

ELEVATION: 1,435'

RESTRICTIONS:

PETS: On leash only

FIRES: In fire rings or grates; check for burn bans

ALCOHOL: Prohibited in all public/ outdoor areas

VEHICLES: 2/site

OTHER: Maximum 8 people/site; guests must leave by 10 p.m.; quiet time 10 p.m.– 6 a.m.; bring your own firewood or charcoal; limited supplies at headquarters; pick up main supplies in Quanah; gathering firewood prohibited

more level, but the outer sites, especially site 29, are set back in the brush for more privacy. Continuing south on the park road, past the showers, is the new Cottonwood camping area, which includes a group tent area with four individual sites. Returning to the main road, turn left and follow that road along the cedar-covered cliff with areas where the water could easily pour over the road in a thunderstorm. At the top of the road, go past the RV area and scenic overlook on your left. Turn right into the Big Pond equestrian camp area just off the pavement. These sites, 37–42, are perched along a canyon with excellent views of the surrounding territory. There are central hitching rails for your horses, but no corrals. On a quiet day, you can easily imagine an early cowboy tending his campfire here while watching the brush for the slightest movement indicating danger. It is also easy to see the Comanche warrior defending this beautiful land, where his ancestors had been at home for many years.

Continuing on the paved road, sites 43–47 and the group area provide some of the premier tent-camping sites in Texas. The group area can also be used as five individual tent sites if not reserved by a group. These breezy wide-open sites sit on a small, elevated peninsula with unrestricted views over the mesas and canyons as far as you can see. They also look down on the Big Pond, where the local birds, deer, coyotes, jackrabbits, and other wildlife meet for life-sustaining water. Be sure to bring binoculars for the best views and a camera for sunsets as spectacular as those enjoyed by the cowboys and Comanches who were here not that long ago.

As you return toward headquarters, turn right into the scenic-view area, where the 2-mile Bull Canyon Hiking Trail is located. Be sure to take water any time of year and watch your step, in case any local reptiles are lounging on the pathway. From the scenic viewpoint, you also look down on Lake Copper Breaks, where there are two additional trails: 0.5-mile Juniper Ridge Nature Trail and Rocky Ledges Loop. Note that the loop also allows mountain bikes.

Whatever your interest, spend some reflective time at this authentic scene of Texas history.

VOICES FROM THE CAMPFIRE AND RECOMMENDED READING

I wish I knew where I was going. Doomed to be "carried of the spirit into the wilderness," I suppose. I wish I could be more moderate in my desires, but cannot, and so there is no rest.
    William Frederic *Badè, The Life and Letters of John Muir,* Vol. I (Boston, Houghton Mifflin Company, 1924).

The white men were grunts, bluecoats, cavalry, and dragoons; mostly veterans of the War Between the States who now found themselves at the edge of the known universe, ascending to the turreted rock towers that gated the fabled Llano Estacado—Coronado's term for it, meaning "palisaded plains" of West Texas, a country populated exclusively by the most hostile Indians on the continents, where few U.S. soldiers had ever gone before. The llano was a place of extreme desolation, a vast trackless, and featureless ocean of grass where white men became lost and disoriented and died of thirst; a place where the imperial Spanish had once marched confidently forth to hunt Comanches, only to find that they themselves were the hunted, the ones to be slaughtered.
    S. C. Gwynne, *Empire of the Summer Moon* (New York, Scribner, 2010).

This Texas legend is not interested in posing for a photo.

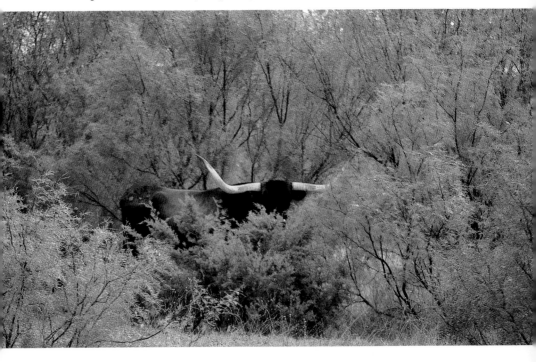

BACKCOUNTRY ADVENTURES

This great park has a nice variety of backcountry trails that allow a mixed use of hiking, biking, and horseback riding. Pick up the detailed trail map and choose your destination. The 1.63-mile Rocky Ledges Loop is a real challenge for both hikers and experienced off-road bikers. The 3.69-mile equestrian trail is a great place to enjoy your trusty mount in an area where both Texas cowboys and local tribes most certainly rode in the not-too-distant past.

BEST LOCAL FOOD AND DRINK

Quanah is a nice town just north of the park. For good food in a historical setting, visit the Medicine Mound Depot (940-663-5619). In nearby Crowell, join the locals who help themselves to a cup of coffee and enjoy a homemade breakfast at Tater's (940-684-1491; taterscafe.com). For a more gourmet treat and fresh cooking, stop by the Home Bakery & Eatery (940-684-1653).

Copper Breaks State Park

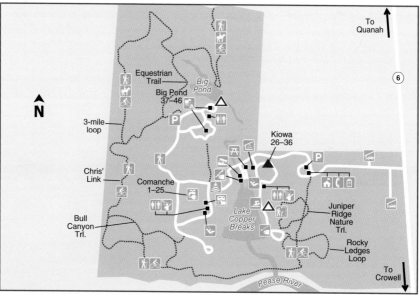

GETTING THERE

From US 287 in Quanah, travel 12.7 miles south on TX 6 to Park Road 62. Turn right. Headquarters is 0.7 mile straight ahead.

GPS COORDINATES: N34° 6.714' W99° 44.586'

36

⚲ Lake Arrowhead State Park

Beauty: ★★★ / Privacy: ★★★ / Spaciousness: ★★★ / Quiet: ★★★ / Security: ★★★★ / Cleanliness: ★★★

Bring your camera and binoculars to scan this area for bird activity.

Located less than 30 minutes from the city of Wichita Falls, this 16,200-acre lake attracts not only fishing enthusiasts from all over North Texas and southern Oklahoma, but also serves as a retreat for Midwestern College students and Sheppard Air Force Base personnel. Especially in the summer, the lake breeze and swimming area are essential to surviving the hot weather made famous by the Hotter'N Hell Hundred bicycle race. There is also a 5.5-mile hike-horse-bike trail for those trying to get a little exercise.

As you leave the entrance station, there is a disc golf course built into a grove of heavy mesquite, which adds to the game's challenge. There is also a modern equestrian campground with four sites that include electricity.

As you return to the main road, the lake appears on the horizon, where sometimes campers will see a red-tailed hawk racing low over the trees looking for lunch. Continue past the day-use area on the right until the road turns toward the lake and sites 61–67. These spacious, level sites are within view of the lake and near the prairie dog town, which is active with these cute—but definitely wild—cousins of the squirrel. The prairie dogs move quickly between mounds but always seem to be wary of hawks or other predators on the hunt. The campsites are also close to the fishing pier and swimming area at the road's end.

Fishing for your own dinner is the way to go . . . for some.

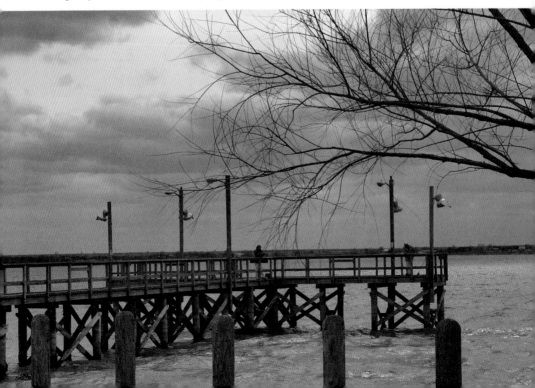

KEY INFORMATION

ADDRESS: 229 Park Road 63, Wichita Falls, TX 76310

CONTACT: 940-528-2211, tpwd.texas.gov /state-parks/lake-arrowhead

OPERATED BY: Texas Parks & Wildlife Department

OPEN: Year-round

SITES: 19 water only; Group Primitive walk-in area (5 sites, 40 person max, 50-yard walk)

EACH SITE: Covered picnic table, fire ring, and water

ASSIGNMENT: First come, first served until site-specific reservation system begins in 2018

REGISTRATION: At headquarters or reserve at texas.reserveworld.com or 512-389-8900

FACILITIES: Restrooms in picnic area, restrooms and showers in RV area, boat ramp, swimming area

PARKING: At each site

FEE: $10/night water-only sites; $7 walk-in sites; $3/person entrance fee, age 12 and under free

ELEVATION: 942'

RESTRICTIONS:

PETS: On leash only

FIRES: In fire rings

ALCOHOL: Prohibited in all public/ outdoor areas

VEHICLES: 2/site

OTHER: Maximum 8 people/site; guests must leave by 10 p.m.; quiet time 10 p.m.– 6 a.m.; bring your own firewood or charcoal; limited supplies at headquarters; pick up main supplies in Wichita Falls; gathering firewood prohibited

Back on the main road, turn right just past site 61 to reach sites 57–60, which are arranged around a circular drive. These well-spaced sites are away from the traffic and have some tree cover. Look for site 59 with its large grass-covered tent pad and a view over the backwater areas of the lake. Bring your camera and binoculars to scan this area for bird activity in the early morning or late afternoon. As you turn right out of the circle, sites 49–56 also line the backwater area but are a little closer together. They are also the tent sites nearest to the modern restrooms and showers in the RV area.

As you leave the park, note the Primitive Group Camping Area Trail for those beginning backpackers and campers preparing for their next trip to wilder parts of Texas or beyond. This 5.5-mile trail allows hikers, mountain bikers, and equestrians. It is moderately strenuous, so be sure to bring sufficient water. Whether you are trying out new hiking boots or a new backpack or just trying to get in shape, this trail is a good fit.

After you hit the trail, return to your campsite, grab your fishing gear or swimsuit, and head to the lake. There is a large protected swimming area just across the grassy area from tent sites 61–67, and next to it is the fishing pier and fish-cleaning station for those crappie, catfish, bass, and perch. The water-skiing crowd will appreciate the nice boat ramp in summer.

Given this lake's location near the edge of the arid West Texas frontier, fill your water bottles, get a big hat and a strong walking stick, and make your reservations early.

VOICES FROM THE CAMPFIRE AND RECOMMENDED READING

Most of my wandering in the desert I've done alone. . . . I generally prefer to go into places where no one else wants to go. I find that in contemplating the natural world my pleasure is greater if there are not too many others contemplating it with me, at the same time. However, there are special hazards in traveling alone. Your chances of dying, in case of sickness or accident, are much improved.

Edward Abbey, *Desert Solitaire: A Season in the Wilderness* (New York, McGraw-Hill, 1968).

BACKCOUNTRY ADVENTURES

After enjoying this nice park, travel south toward Jacksboro and Fort Richardson State Park, Historic Site & Lost Creek Reservoir State Trailway. The restored frontier buildings and exhibits give a fascinating look into a period of Texas history when the battle between European settlers and American Indians was a true war. There are primitive tent sites, and the 10-mile Lost Creek Reservoir State Trailway is part of the Rails-to-Trails Conservancy program.

BEST LOCAL FOOD AND DRINK

You'll find an array of eating choices in nearby Wichita Falls, including BackPorch Drafthouse (940-234-7777; bpdrafthouse.com) for good food, service, and draft beer in a family-friendly atmosphere. Pelican's (940-687-0072; pelicansurfclub.com) offers wonderful seafood. A visit to El Mejicano (940-322-1846; elmejicanorestaurant.com), Gutierrez (940-322-3511), or Casa Mañana (940-723-5661) for Mexican food will fill you up before hitting the trail.

Lake Arrowhead State Park

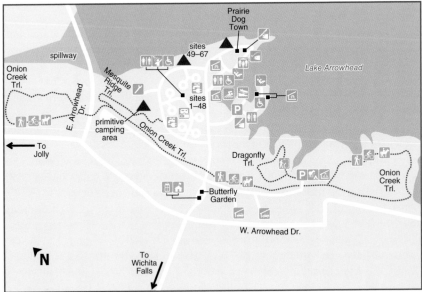

GETTING THERE

From the intersection of US 281 and US 287 in Wichita Falls, take US 281 S and drive 5 miles. Turn left onto FM 1954. The park entrance is 7.6 miles straight ahead.

GPS COORDINATES: N33° 45.498' W98° 23.682'

37

Palo Duro Canyon State Park

Beauty: ★★★★ / Privacy: ★★★ / Spaciousness: ★★★ / Quiet: ★★★ / Security: ★★★★ / Cleanliness: ★★★

Surrounding cliffs of bright red claystone, white gypsum, and yellow, gray, and lavender mudstone will keep photographers busy until the last rays of sundown.

As you travel the Panhandle of Texas, the horizons seem limitless and cotton fields surround you in every direction. However, approaching the entrance of this popular park, the first-time visitor will be pleasantly surprised, if not a little awestruck, by the massive canyon that opens up before you here. Stretching 120 miles and up to 800 feet deep, this geological marvel was formed by the seemingly peaceful Prairie Dog Town Fork of the Red River, which crosses the park road at six different places and provides nice wading spots and even a mud bath or two for visitors. At most times of the year, you can cross safely on foot or by car, but a quick look at the flood gauge and the amount of sand piled up by a park bulldozer is a reminder that water is a powerful and dangerous force to be respected.

Leaving the entrance station and descending into the canyon, the scenic overlook and trailhead to the Civilian Conservation Corps Trail is 0.8 mile on your right along with the turnoff to the visitor center and gift shop. Proceeding 2.1 miles down the switchback roadway, you reach the Pioneer Amphitheater, where the outdoor musical extravaganza *Texas* has been playing for more than four decades to packed audiences during cool summer evenings. This classic attraction of the Texas Panhandle uses the canyon beauty as a backdrop and is a tradition with many locals and travelers alike. The production has been musically reproduced, and during the performance, Feldman's Wrong Way Diner provides food to hungry hikers and campers wishing to complete their Texas experience.

High canyon walls keep the uncivilized city world away.

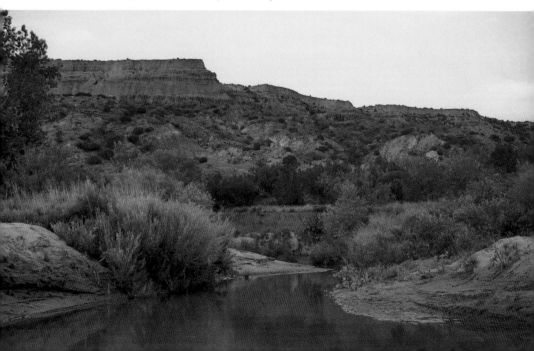

KEY INFORMATION

ADDRESS: 11450 TX Park Road 5, Canyon, TX 79015

CONTACT: 806-488-2227 or 806-488-2506, tpwd.texas.gov/state-parks /palo-duro-canyon

OPERATED BY: Texas Parks & Wildlife Department

OPEN: Year-round

SITES: 25 tent sites in Cactus, Fortress Cliff areas

EACH SITE: Covered picnic table, fire pit

ASSIGNMENT: First come, first served until site-specific reservation system begins in 2018

REGISTRATION: At headquarters or reserve at texas.reserveworld.com or 512-389-8900

FACILITIES: Restrooms and showers near tent areas, visitor center, park store, stables, amphitheater, sponsored youth group tent site

PARKING: At each site

FEE: $16; $5/person entrance fee, age 12 and under free

ELEVATION: 3,450'

RESTRICTIONS:

PETS: On leash only

FIRES: In fire pits (check with park for any burn bans in effect)

ALCOHOL: Prohibited in all public/ outdoor areas

VEHICLES: 2/site

OTHER: Maximum 8 people/site; guests must leave by 10 p.m.; quiet time 10 p.m.– 6 a.m.; bring your own firewood or charcoal; limited supplies at park store located at The Trading Post; pick up main supplies in Canyon or Amarillo; gathering firewood prohibited

Returning to the main park road, travel 3.2 miles to the Fortress Cliff Camp Area on the right. As you enter the campground, look for sites 49, 47, 45, 43, and 41 backing up to the heavy canyon vegetation. This tent-site area has excellent views of the surrounding cliffs of bright red claystone and white gypsum, along with yellow, gray, and lavender mudstone— all of which will keep the photographers in your group busy until the last rays of a sunset

After miles of flat cotton fields, these first views are the best kind of surprise.

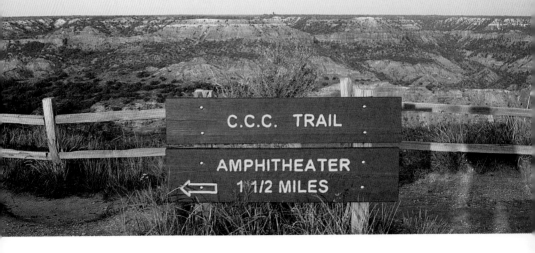

disappear behind the canyon rim and the western horizon. With the coming of nighttime, be sure to enjoy the dark skies and the intoxicating smell of a wood fire, which is finally allowed after a summer of burn bans in many Texas parks.

Turning right out of Fortress Cliff, proceed 1.4 miles to the Cactus Camp Area and sites 70–76. The park road runs down the middle of these sites and is 0.4 mile before the large Mesquite Camp Area, which has modern restrooms and showers, but is also very popular with RVers and mountain bikers setting up weekend base camp.

While camping at Palo Duro State Park, there are multiple options for outdoor adventure and exercise, including hiking, horseback riding on equestrian trails, mountain biking, and even running on a rugged 11-mile trail for the more recent athletic pioneer. For a unique view, hike part of the new Comanche Trail, which goes along the canyon wall on the east side of the road.

From the Mesquite Camp Area, travel the final 0.8 mile to the road's end and the historical marker for the Red River War. This 1874 battle led to the capture of some 1,400 horses that belonged to various American Indian tribes who had lived and hunted buffalo on the high plains for multiple generations. The loss of the horses forced the tribes back to the reservations in Oklahoma and allowed Charles Goodnight to eventually run 100,000 head of cattle in the Palo Duro Canyon area. When a large group of Comanches and Kiowas returned in 1878, they found no buffalo remaining and settled for a treaty that allowed them to receive two beef cattle a day until they returned to their reservations, thus ending the era of traditional hunting by the tribes and beginning the legend of the trail drive and the Texas Cowboy.

VOICES FROM THE CAMPFIRE AND RECOMMENDED READING

Letter of Chief Seathl (Seattle) of the Suwamish Tribe to the President of the United States of America, Franklin Pierce, 1854

. . . One thing we know, which the white man may one day discover—our God is the same God. You may think now that you own Him as you wish to own our land: but you cannot. He is the God of man; and his compassion is equal for the red man and the white. This earth is precious to Him and to harm the earth is to heap contempt on its Creator. The whites too shall pass; perhaps sooner than all other tribes. Continue to contaminate your bed, and you will one night suffocate in your own waste.

Ed McGaa, Eagle Man, Mother Earth Spirituality (New York, HarperCollins, 1990).

BACKCOUNTRY ADVENTURES

The sheer size of Palo Duro Canyon allows the tent camper to hike, bike, ride, or even run on a variety of trails. Even on crowded weekends, you can get away with just a little effort. On weekdays, it's a great outdoor experience, especially if you are a local resident or college student whose hometown or campus might be a little topographically challenged.

BEST LOCAL FOOD AND DRINK

The city of Canyon is fairly close to the park entrance. Try the Ranch House Cafe (806-655-8785; theranchhousecafe.com) for breakfast, lunch at Rockin' Zebra Soda Shoppe

(806-655-3381) for great sandwiches and ice cream in an old soda shop atmosphere, or lunch/dinner at Fat-Boys Bar-B-Que (806-655-7363) or Feldman's (806-655-1800; feldmansdiner.com), great American food and trains running overhead—very family oriented. Pepito's (806-655-4736) will handle a Tex-Mex fix.

Amarillo is to the northwest and contains a true Texas tradition: The Big Texan Steak Ranch (806-372-6000; bigtexan.com), a genuine tourist attraction, serving up traditional Texas fare in a Wild West atmosphere that even Hollywood or Disney World couldn't match.

Palo Duro Canyon State Park

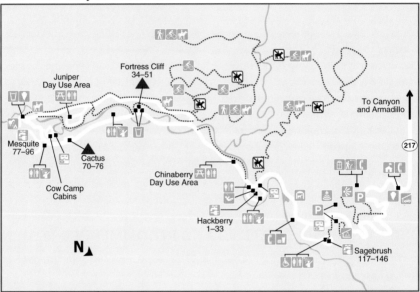

GETTING THERE

From I-25 in Canyon, 12 miles south of Amarillo, proceed 14 miles east on TX 217 to the entrance station and Park Road 5.

GPS COORDINATES: N34° 59.052' W101° 42.120'

DEEP EAST TEXAS AND THE BIG THICKET

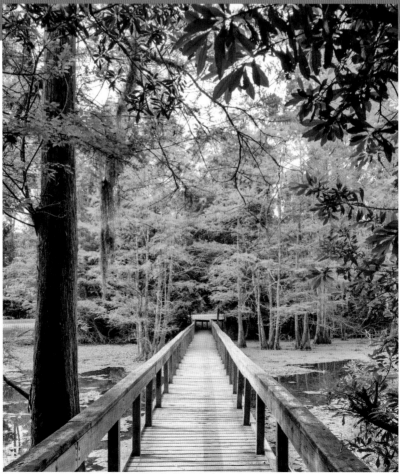

Photo credit: *Shutterstock*

A walkway to paradise (Martin Dies, Jr. State Park; see page 153)

38

Fairfield Lake State Park

Beauty: ★★★ / Privacy: ★★★ / Spaciousness: ★★★★ / Quiet: ★★★★ / Security: ★★★ / Cleanliness: ★★★

Once settled in to your site, grab the fishing gear for a wide range of catches.

If you are looking for a hidden piece of Texas wilderness that offers great fishing, hiking, horseback riding, and tent camping without an RV in sight, Fairfield Lake State Park is your destination. Only 8 miles off I-45, the terrain here is a mix of hill country and Deep East Texas, where sleek vultures are often flying high overhead looking for lunch.

As you approach the entrance station, the Dockery Trail is on the right and parking for the Big Brown Creek Primitive Camping Area is on the left. This 6-mile trail allows hiking, mountain bikes, and horses, and it ends at primitive tent sites near the lake.

Returning to the main road, enter the park and travel straight ahead on PW 5078 for 1.4 miles past the Fairfield Lake Bird-Watching Trail on the left. Continue another 1.6 miles to the Springfield Camping Area on your left, where you will find 35 tent sites shaded by huge oak trees. These well-spaced sites line both sides of the road, with sites 14, 16, 18, and 20 backing up to deep forest and offering a feeling of remoteness. Sites 22, 23, 26, 28, and 29 have water views and even prime frontage, depending on the water level. Combined with centrally located restrooms and showers for this tent-only campground, you have a relaxed base for the weekend. (Note: site numbers may change after recent construction is completed.)

Note that this popular tent campground is closed yearly from around mid-December until the end of February or so. Be sure to call ahead for reservations and exact opening

A wide-open nature trail will help you forget the crowded interstate from which you just escaped.

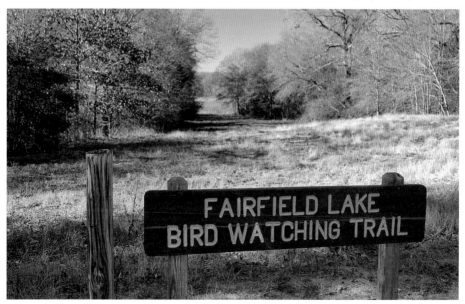

KEY INFORMATION

ADDRESS: 123 State Park Road 64, Fairfield, TX 75840

CONTACT: 903-389-4514, tpwd.texas.gov/state-parks/fairfield-lake

OPERATED BY: Texas Parks & Wildlife Department

OPEN: Year-round

SITES: 33 water only

EACH SITE: Picnic table, fire ring, lantern hook

ASSIGNMENT: First come, first served until site-specific reservation system begins in 2018

REGISTRATION: At headquarters or reserve at texas.reserveworld.com or 512-389-8900

FACILITIES: Modern restrooms and showers

PARKING: At each site

FEE: $12 water-only sites; $9 primitive camping; $4/person entrance fee, $2 age 65 and older, free for those under age 13 and over age 79

ELEVATION: 362'

RESTRICTIONS:

PETS: On leash only

FIRES: In fire rings only; check for burn bans

ALCOHOL: Prohibited in all public/outdoor areas

VEHICLES: 2/site

OTHER: Maximum 8 people/site; guests must leave by 10 p.m.; quiet time 10 p.m.–6 a.m.; bring your own firewood or charcoal; limited supplies at park store; main supplies in Fairfield; gathering firewood prohibited

---

dates. Also, the entire Springfield and Post Oak loops may be closed for road construction projects in 2018.

As you return to the main road, a left turn takes you to two large camping areas that have not only electricity but also level tent pads perfect for the local Boy Scout troop. Look for sites 91 and 93 for some privacy and easy access to a short trail connecting it to Springfield.

Once settled at your site, grab the fishing gear for a wide range of catches, including red drum, crappie, blue tilapia, largemouth bass, and that Texas favorite, channel catfish (limit 25/day, please). If not fishing, grab a good book, sit back, relax, and enjoy this peaceful park, where the main sounds you hear are the birds and the wind.

When you are ready for some exercise, try Big Brown Creek Trail, which starts in the upland region of the Post Oak Savannah Ecoregion of Texas and ends 2.5 miles later in the flood plain of Big Brown Creek. You'll pass under towering post oaks, blackjack oaks, water oaks, and black hickory and move alongside eastern red cedars, yaupons, holly, and American beautyberry as you descend to the creek. As you near the trail's end, look for the primitive camping area if you wish to leave the comforts of the car-camping area behind. A flush toilet and potable water are available for those who choose to visit this wilder portion of the park. Keep in mind that this trail and the tent areas can be pretty muddy after heavy rain, and they are closed from December through February each year.

The other trail is Dockery Trail, which follows the perimeter of the park and is also open to hikers, bikers, and equestrians. It also leaves from the parking lot just outside the park entrance and eventually leads to the lake some 6 miles later. If you have any energy left, the 2-mile nature walk and 1-mile bird-watching trail are good ways to finish your day and send you back to your campsite ready for a cold drink and that good book you left unfinished.

Although not well known outside the region, this park is very popular, so make your reservations early.

VOICES FROM THE CAMPFIRE AND RECOMMENDED READING

The Parker raid marked the moment in history when the westernmost tendrils of the nascent American empire touched the easternmost tip of a vast, primitive, and equally lethal inland empire dominated by the Comanche Indians. No one understood this at the time. . . . Neither the Americans nor the Indians they confronted along that raw frontier had the remotest idea of the other's geographical size or military power. Both, as it turned out, had for the past two centuries been busily engaged in the bloody conquest and near-extermination of Native American tribes. Both had succeeded in hugely expanding the lands under their control. The difference was that the Comanches were content with what they had won. The Anglo-Americans, children of Manifest Destiny, were not. Now, at this lonely spot by the Navasota River, the relentless American drive westward had finally brought them together. The meaning of their meeting, and the moment itself, became completely clear only in hindsight.

S. C. Gwynne, *Empire of the Summer Moon* (New York, Scribner, 2010).

Fellow-citizens, I will not enlarge further on your national inconsistencies. The existence of slavery in this country brands your republicanism as a sham, your humanity as a base pretense, and your Christianity as a lie. It destroys your moral power abroad; it corrupts your politicians at home. It saps the foundation of religion, it makes your name a hissing and a bye-word to a mocking earth. It is the antagonistic force in your government, the only thing that seriously disturbs and endangers your Union.

Frederick Douglass on Slavery and the Civil War (Mineola, NY, Dover Publications, 2003).

BACKCOUNTRY ADVENTURES

Just a short drive to the west of Fairfield is the town of Mexia and three areas worth visiting. The first two are Old Fort Parker and Fort Parker State Park, where the Navasota River has been a water source for many an early Texas pioneer, including the family of Cynthia Ann Parker, whose kidnapping by Comanches sparked an entire legend. This heavily wooded and well-maintained state park contains 10 secluded tent sites and more than 11 miles of trails, and it is a great starting point for a leisurely canoe or kayak trip on the Navasota River between the park and the Confederate Reunion Grounds. The third area is the Confederate Reunion Grounds State Historic Site. Beginning in the 1880s, Camp 94 of the United Confederate Veterans began holding reunions, which attracted as many as 7,000 people from all over Texas "to perpetuate the memories of our fallen comrades, to administer to the wants of those who were permanently disabled in the service, and to aid the indigent widows and orphans of deceased Confederate soldiers, to preserve and maintain that sentiment of fraternity born of the hardships and dangers shared in the march, bivouac and the battlefield" (1889 Constitution of Camp 94 UCV).

While the number of Civil War battles on Texas soil was small, the number of Texan soldiers sacrificed on the battlefields was large, all for the lost cause of the Confederacy and secession opposed by many Texans, including Governor Sam Houston. At this historic site, take a backcountry adventure in time to try to understand the Civil War and how it still affects our cultural relations in a state that's more diverse now than ever.

BEST LOCAL FOOD AND DRINK

If you're really hungry after a long hike, stop in longtime family-run Sam's Original Restaurant (903-389-7267; samsoriginal.com). Order a little something off the menu or enjoy the all-you-can-eat buffet. Choices range from salads to barbecue and Southern home cooking. If you don't arrive too late, there's homemade pie to top off the meal, or order a whole pie ahead of time to take home. Padrinos (903-389-5282; fairfieldpadrinos.com) is also family owned and offers wonderful made-from-scratch Italian dishes and pizza. For a summer treat, stop at one of the roadside stands near the interstate for homegrown peaches.

Fairfield Lake State Park

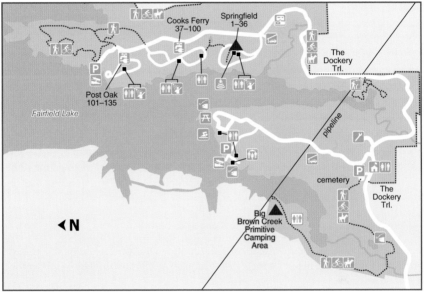

GETTING THERE

From the intersection of I-45 and US 84 in Fairfield, take US 84 W 1.4 miles. Turn left onto Ranch Road 488 and drive 1.7 miles. Keep right to continue onto FM 2570 N/ Ranch Road 1124 and drive 1.3 miles. Turn right onto FM 3285 and drive 3.1 miles; the park entrance is straight ahead.

GPS COORDINATES: N31° 45.900' W96° 4.368'

39

⚠ Huntsville State Park

Beauty: ★★★★ / Privacy: ★★★ / Spaciousness: ★★★ / Quiet: ★★★ / Security: ★★★ / Cleanliness: ★★★

Huntsville State Park is a piece of wilderness hidden from the big city.

As you search the state for that special camping spot, parks located just off the interstate system are generally not your first choice. However, this popular park has a large tent-camping area hidden in the tall pines and overlooking the scenic shores of Lake Raven. Just south of Huntsville and north of outer Houston suburbia, this region of the piney woods of East Texas and the Sam Houston National Forest is a close-in park not to be missed.

Turning west off of I-45, Park Road 40 takes you 1.3 miles into heavy tree cover and quickly leaves the speeding traffic world behind. Signs for DEER CROSSING and ALLIGATORS EXIST IN THE PARK confirm you have left the human habitat and entered an island of wilderness.

As you leave the entrance station, turn left on Park Road 40A toward Coloneh/Raven Hill Camping Areas. With towering pine trees shading the way, go past the Raven Hill RV area and turn right into sites 47–59. The lake quickly appears on your right, and premium waterfront sites 57–60 have not only clear views of the water but also reflections of spectacular sunset colors behind the distant tree-lined shore.

Continue to the right for more premium waterfront sites 62–64 and 67–72, which will fill up quickly. However, even if full, the interior sites are sufficiently elevated for you to still enjoy the lake. Travel farther into the Coloneh Camping Area past the fishing pier on your

A true refuge from the urban cement jungle; photo credit: *Shutterstock*

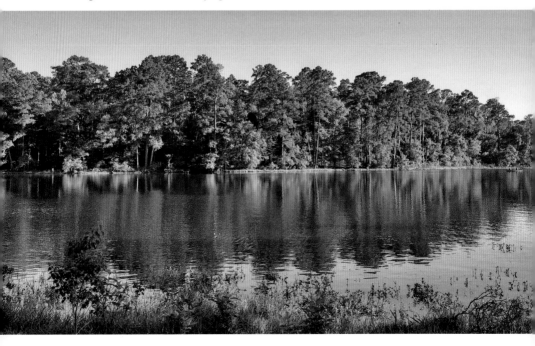

KEY INFORMATION

ADDRESS: 565 Park Road 40 W, Huntsville, TX 77340

CONTACT: 936-295-5644, tpwd.texas.gov/state-parks/huntsville

OPERATED BY: Texas Parks & Wildlife Department

OPEN: Year-round

SITES: 87

EACH SITE: Picnic table, fire ring, lantern hook, central water

ASSIGNMENT: First come, first served until site-specific reservation system begins in 2018

REGISTRATION: At headquarters or reserve at texas.reserveworld.com or 512-389-8900

FACILITIES: Modern restrooms and showers, boat rentals, nature center

PARKING: At each site

FEE: $15; $5/person entrance fee, age 12 and under free

ELEVATION: 432'

RESTRICTIONS:

PETS: On leash only

FIRES: In fire rings

ALCOHOL: Prohibited in all public/outdoor areas

VEHICLES: 2/site

OTHER: Maximum 8 people/site; guests must leave by 10 p.m.; quiet time 10 p.m.–6 a.m.; bring your own firewood or charcoal; limited supplies at park store; pick up main supplies in Huntsville; gathering firewood prohibited

right for another 14 waterfront tent sites with modern restrooms and showers in the circle area. There is also trailhead parking for 13 miles of hiking and biking trails.

Returning to the main road, turn left toward the bathhouse buildings, built by one of the few African American companies of the Civilian Conservation Corps (CCC). At this popular day-use spot, you can rent canoes, kayaks, and flat-bottom boats. Horseback riding is no longer offered or allowed on trails.

After setting up your tent, begin your exploration at the nature center immediately next to the entrance station. This small but functional center has exhibits about the varied plant life you will encounter on the trail system, including loblolly and shortleaf pines towering over dogwoods flowering in the spring. The park has allowed most of the understory to remain quite thick and wild enough to hide fox, opossums, white-tailed deer, and it's wet enough for an occasional alligator.

Trailhead parking is across the street from the nature center and makes an excellent place to begin your hike. The trail is only moderately difficult but it does require sufficient water and snacks if you plan to head deep into the red maples, dogwoods, and sassafras listening for pileated woodpeckers. As always, stay on the marked trail to avoid damaging the ecosystem or encountering a healthy patch of poison ivy.

Returning to the main road, continue approximately 1 mile to the park's day-use area for a protected swimming area with a bathhouse on your left. This area is very popular in warm weather and also offers canoe, kayak, and flat-bottom boat rentals. The nearby park store offers drinks, snacks, basic camping supplies, and outdoor items.

VOICES FROM THE CAMPFIRE AND RECOMMENDED READING

A question that will be asked is why I am willing to teach non-Indians about Native American spirituality and about my own spiritual experiences. . . . We do not have any choice. It is one world that we live in. If the Native Americans keep all their spirituality within their own community, the old wisdom that has performed so well will not be allowed to work its environmental medicine on the world where it is desperately needed.

Global warming, acid rain, overpopulation, and deforestation are real. It is a mess, and all of us two-leggeds will have to work together to get ourselves out of it.

Ed McGaa, Eagle Man, Mother Earth Spirituality (New York, HarperCollins, 1990).

BACKCOUNTRY ADVENTURES

Pick up the excellent detailed trail map at the entrance station and choose from nearly 20 miles of trails, including the 6.8-mile Chinquapin Trail and the 8.5-mile Triple C Trail honoring the CCC work in the park. You can also connect to the Lone Star Trailhead and the 129-mile Sam Houston National Forest trail system.

BEST LOCAL FOOD AND DRINK

Nearby Huntsville has a wide range of food choices, including Farmhouse Cafe (936-435-1450), Five Loaves Deli (936-439-9400; fiveloavesdeli.com), and Bennie J's Smoke Pit (936-439-9559).

Huntsville State Park

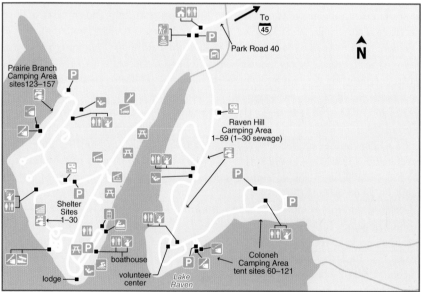

GETTING THERE

From Huntsville, drive 8 miles south on I-45, then 1.3 miles west on PR 40.

GPS COORDINATES: N30° 37.698' W95° 31.566'

40

⛺ Martin Dies, Jr. State Park

Beauty: ★★★★ / Privacy: ★★★ / Spaciousness: ★★★ / Quiet: ★★★ / Security: ★★★★ / Cleanliness: ★★★★

Here you'll get a close-up view of one of the premier natural areas in the country, where you might see alligators, roadrunners, and numerous deer appearing like ghosts out of the dense underbrush at sunset.

Located on the northern edge of the Big Thicket, this Deep East Texas park combines the best of open waters on B. A. Steinhagen Reservoir and extensive wilderness swamp areas. You can rent canoes or bring your own boat for a close-up view of one of the premier natural areas in the country, where you might see alligators, roadrunners, and numerous deer appearing like ghosts out of the dense underbrush at sunset.

As you approach on US 190, the park is split into the Hen House Ridge Unit to the south and the Walnut Ridge Unit to the north. The main headquarters is to the south of Park Road 48, at the entrance to the Hen House Ridge Unit. Continue straight over the bridge, where you get your first good look at the rugged backwater of the Gum Slough, until you reach

Sunset and sunrise views are the tent camper's best reward.

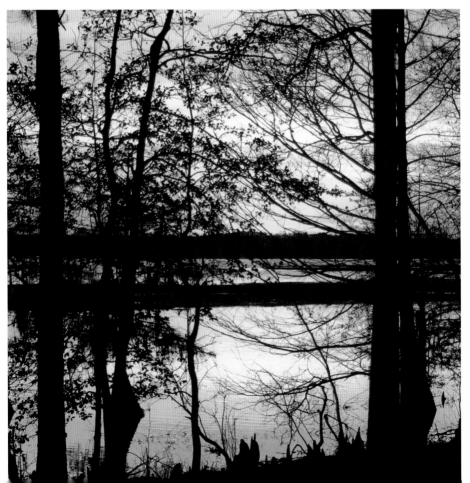

KEY INFORMATION

ADDRESS: 634 Park Road 48 S, Jasper, TX 75951

CONTACT: 409-384-5231, tpwd.texas.gov/state-parks/martin-dies-jr

OPERATED BY: Texas Parks & Wildlife Department

OPEN: Year-round

SITES: 51 (changing—see note on p. 155)

EACH SITE: Picnic table

ASSIGNMENT: First come, first served until site-specific reservation system begins in 2018

REGISTRATION: At headquarters or reserve at texas.reserveworld.com or 512-389-8900

FACILITIES: Restrooms and showers; boat ramps; fishing pier; bike, canoe, and kayak rentals

PARKING: At each site

FEE: $14; $4/person entrance fee, $2 for seniors, age 12 and under free

ELEVATION: 90'

RESTRICTIONS:

PETS: On leash only

FIRES: In fire rings or grills only

ALCOHOL: Prohibited in all public/outdoor areas

VEHICLES: 2/site

OTHER: Maximum 8 people/site; guests must leave by 10 p.m.; quiet time 10 p.m.–6 a.m.; bring your own charcoal; limited supplies at park store or from park host (firewood only); pick up main supplies in Jasper or Zavalla

---

premier waterfront tent-camping sites 36–38 and 39–45. The views here are great and have a protected swimming area nearby in the day-use area. The interior sites are a little larger and still have a lake view with room to spread out in the grassy meadow. Turning the corner away from the lake leads to the interior sites 67–79, in case the other sites are not available.

Big Thicket wildlife in a small package; photo credit: *Shutterstock*

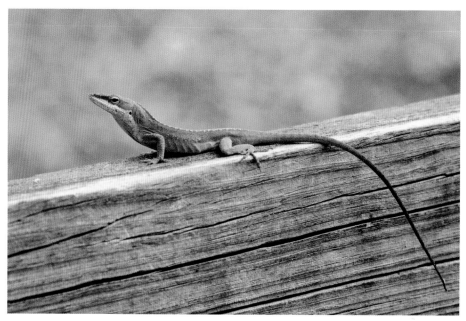

Returning toward headquarters, don't miss the 2.2-mile slough trail on your right for great photography spots and solitude. Note that this trail returns to PR 48 just a short distance from the 1.1-mile Forest Trail, so take along water and keep a sharp lookout for any resident reptiles that might be using the trail at the same time as you. If you don't want to go alone, there are guided interpretive walks from the headquarters.

Back in your auto, return to US 190, turn left, and then make an immediate right turn on North PR 48 toward the Walnut Ridge Unit. While you will want to visit the Nature Center, the Wildscape Herb Garden, and the 1.5-mile Wildlife Trail, the real attraction is the wilderness feel of hanging moss and the low-water sloughs near the roadway. At 0.7 mile past the entrance station, make a right turn and park in the Walnut Slough Day Use area for access to the 0.8-mile Island Trail and a long boardwalk connecting to the 0.4-mile Loop Trail, which provides excellent sunrise and sunset photography and bird-watching opportunities.

Returning to the main road, go past the shelter area and turn right on the one-way road toward sites 105–182. Site 107 on your far right is in the RV area but provides a perfect sunset view over the water. Continue through the RV area to tent sites 125–132. Huge trees shade this area, and site 125 has the lake on one side and the slough on the other. Sites 126–132 back up to the slough for that up-close experience of the Big Thicket.

Note: As of publication date, site numbers for this entire park were being renumbered. Check the park website or call the park office for updated site references.

Leaving the park, head south to the patchwork of wilderness areas that make up the 100,000-acre Big Thicket National Preserve. Start at the visitor center on US 69 south of Woodville and bring your hiking boots, cameras, and day packs to enjoy more than 45 miles of hiking trails and a unique mix of plants—such as cacti and yucca plants—that coexist with the swamps and cypress trees.

While in the Big Thicket area, check out Village Creek State Park for some hidden but first-class tent-camping opportunities. The walk-in sites were previously closed due to flood damage, so be sure to contact the park ahead of time to determine availability. Despite the hurricanes, which have hammered this already wild and untamed portion of Deep East Texas, this park still offers paddling experiences on marked paddling trails, the wide-open lake, and the free-flowing tributary of the Neches River, whose very existence is threatened by the large urban area's thirst for another reservoir site.

VOICES FROM THE CAMPFIRE AND RECOMMENDED READING

It really is no exaggeration to say that the Big Thicket is the Biological Crossroads of North America. It contains both temperate and subtropical plants and animals, along with many from the dry, treeless west. In the Thicket there are many varieties of orchids; but there are also species of sagebrush and cacti. In few other places will one find roadrunners alongside alligators, mesquite and yucca alongside cypress and water tupelo.

Pete A. Y. Gunter, *The Big Thicket: An Ecological Reevaluation* (Denton, University of North Texas Press, 1993).

My first real feeling of unease for the natural world I knew came during the early 1950s when the effluent from the big paper mill at Lufkin began turning the Angelina River a putrid black every summer. During the hot, dry low-water months, the river's natural khaki-colored waters were overwhelmed by thousands of gallons of black broth discharged into it by the mill. The word we heard was that this stuff the mill was pumping into the river was harmless. No one I knew dreamed of questioning the mill's right to alter the characteristics of the river, and many naively believed that business and industry would never consider releasing anything harmful into the water or air.

Richard M. Donovan, *Paddling the Wild Neches* (College Station, Texas A&M University Press, 2006).

BACKCOUNTRY ADVENTURES

This park provides a nice mix of interpretive programs, including ranger-led walks and canoe trips down the Angelina River. You can rent single-speed bicycles, canoes, and kayaks to explore this diverse ecosystem. About 5 miles of hiking trails provide up close contact with nature and solitude.

BEST LOCAL FOOD AND DRINK

In Jasper, enjoy home cooking, seafood, and pie at Cedar Tree (409-384-8832); catfish and hushpuppies at The Catfish Cabin (409-384-2228); and home cooking and friendly atmosphere at Elijah's Cafe (409-384-9000).

Martin Dies, Jr. State Park

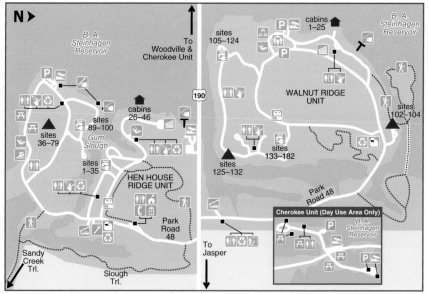

GETTING THERE

From Jasper, travel 10 miles west on US 190. From Woodville, travel 15 miles east on US 190. Park Road 48 is on both sides of the road.

GPS COORDINATES: N30° 50.784' W94° 9.948'

41

Sam Rayburn Reservoir: RAYBURN PARK

Beauty: ★★★★ / Privacy: ★★★ / Spaciousness: ★★★ / Quiet: ★★★ / Security: ★★★ / Cleanliness: ★★★★

These spacious sites follow the shoreline for premium waterfront camping and 180-degree views.

For tent campers who pour over their maps and search out little-known roads leading to the most remote locations, Rayburn Park is a must-stop. Leaving Pineland on FM 83 West, cross the Ayish Bayou and enter the Angelina National Forest. Take FM 705 south into the towering pines and notice the various hunting clubs on your left hanging onto the remaining wildlands threatened by the clear-cutters.

A right turn on South Spur 3127 and then a left on South Spur 3127 qualifies as being officially off the tourist route, but the location is a great tent campground. After you pass the gatehouse and visit with the friendly staff, the first right leads to tent sites 1–10 in the shelter of huge pine trees and lake views on both sides of the road. Check out sites 2, 3, and 4 if you want a personal boat ramp. The other sites are quieter in summer season.

Returning to the main road, continue to the end, veering right for the RV area with new modern restrooms, showers, and awe-inspiring sunset views over the 114,000-acre lake. Veer left for tent-camping sites 55–65. These spacious sites follow the shoreline for premium waterfront camping and 180-degree views. Site 60 is the group tent site. Continue around the corner, and site 65 on the end has maximum privacy and tree cover plus a little shelter on windy days. After leaving this park, don't forget to visit the other U.S. Army Corps of Engineers parks located around the 750 miles of shoreline. Tent campers will find two excellent choices: Twin Dikes and Ebenezer. Both of these parks are located off FM 255

Leave that ski boat at the big boy toy store; get a kayak or canoe to really be human.

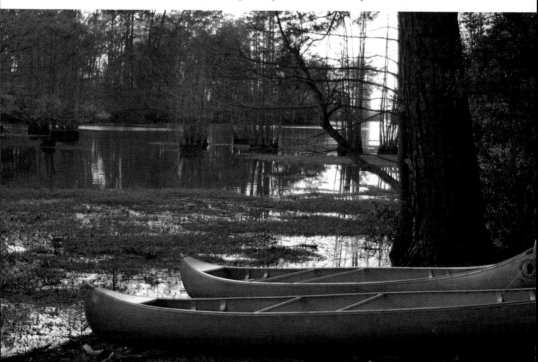

KEY INFORMATION

ADDRESS: Rayburn Park, South Spur 3127, Jasper, TX 75951

CONTACT: 409-384-5716, samrayburn.com /camping-rayburn-park/93; reservations: 877-444-6777, recreation.gov

OPERATED BY: U.S. Army Corps of Engineers

OPEN: Year-round (some tent sites closed during off season)

SITES: 21 nonelectric, 2 tents/site; 1 nonelectric group site (20 person max)

EACH SITE: Picnic table, fire ring, central water

ASSIGNMENT: Reservations (site specific) required online or by phone, on arrival if not made in advance. No staff at gatehouse

REGISTRATION: Park host will come to your site to verify reservation

FACILITIES: Modern restrooms and showers in RV area, vault restrooms in tent-camping areas, boat ramp

PARKING: At each site

FEE: $14, $28 for group site

ELEVATION: 301'

RESTRICTIONS:

PETS: On leash only

FIRES: In fire rings only; check on burn bans

ALCOHOL: Prohibited

VEHICLES: 2/site

OTHER: Maximum 8 people/site; guests must leave by 10 p.m.; quiet time 10 p.m.– 6 a.m.; bring your own firewood or charcoal; no park store; pick up main supplies in Pineland; gathering firewood prohibited

---

on the south side of the reservoir. Whichever park you choose, enjoy yourself in the towering East Texas pines and on the water.

As you travel around this massive reservoir, you soon learn that timber is a crop to the local timber companies, and conflicts with conservationists are not easily resolved. The good news is that sport hunters and fishermen have now realized that the harvesting of trees and the bulldozers that follow are destroying the wildlife they depend on. Without habitat protection, the fish, deer, and game birds will eventually disappear. Tent campers have long known that clear-cutting is a threat to not only wildlife but also the very wilderness they search for as a place of solitude. With the new alliances between the traditional hunting, fishing, and conservation groups, there is some hope that major wilderness areas will be saved.

Returning to your campsite, pull up a chair and read a good book or simply gaze on the seemingly endless miles of waterway. You can also launch your canoe or kayak for a closer inspection of the shoreline, but beware high winds if you venture out too far. Of course, if you brought your sailboat, Sam Rayburn Reservoir will reward you with many hours of wide-open cruising, powered by nature, and leaving no footprints

VOICES FROM THE CAMPFIRE AND RECOMMENDED READING

A clearcut looks like a war zone. It is the radical surgery of the timber business. The soil washes off like blood.

Edward C. Fritz, *Clearcutting: A Crime Against Nature* (Burnet, TX, Eakin Press, 1989).

But beauty is only brain deep. Old-growth and intermediate communities have other values, as well. They serve as living museums to educate present and future generations on the natural heritage of their region. They provide authentic laboratories where scientists may engage in research on such vital subjects as survival and evolution. And they constitute gene pools for substances and products useful to humankind.

Edward C. Fritz, *Realms of Beauty: A Guide to the Wilderness Areas of East Texas* (Austin, University of Texas Press, 1993).

BACKCOUNTRY ADVENTURES

This body of water is big enough to qualify as a wilderness experience. While the reservoir does get more boat traffic on weekends, it is far enough away from the big metropolitan areas to allow some solitude on the water. You can rent kayaks at numerous places, including Lake Boat Rental, Powell Park Resort & Marina, and Soaring Eagle Boat Rentals. There are also guide services to find that perfect fishing spot.

BEST LOCAL FOOD AND DRINK

This massive reservoir is located in a triangle of Lufkin, San Augustine, and Jasper. While Lufkin is the largest town in the area, good food can be found in Jasper at The Catfish Cabin (409-384-2228) and The Catfish Hut (409-384-8017). Hamburger Depot (409-384-5824; hamburgerdepot.com) is also a good choice. If you want something closer, the restaurant at Powell Park Marina (409-584-2624; powellpark.com) has a nice menu and good hamburgers.

Sam Rayburn Reservoir: Rayburn Park

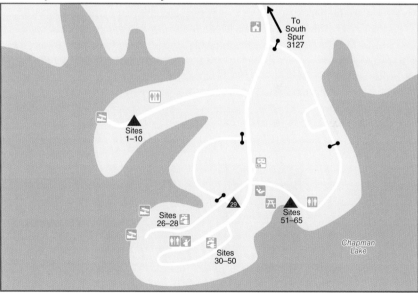

GETTING THERE

From Pineland, travel 22 miles west on FM 83. Turn left onto FM 705 and travel 11 miles. Turn right onto South Spur 3127 and drive 1.5 miles, then turn left into the park entrance.

GPS COORDINATES: N31° 6.618' W94° 6.414'

42

Toledo Bend Reservoir:

INDIAN MOUNDS CAMPGROUND

Beauty: ★★★★ / Privacy: ★★★ / Spaciousness: ★★★ / Quiet: ★★★ / Security: ★★★ / Cleanliness: ★★★

This is rustic tent camping at its best.

As you travel 7 miles east from Hemphill on Farm Road 83, a right turn on Farm Road 3382 leads to a dense forest drive running along the border of the 11,037-acre Indian Mounds Wilderness Area. This rugged part of the Sabine National Forest prohibits any motorized access, and only hikers or equestrian riders may enter the area. Backpacking and primitive camping are also allowed, but do be careful in hunting season.

After the pay station, the road narrows and the trees form a canopy down the long hill toward the water. Deep ravines on both sides are filled with flowering redbuds and dogwoods. A right turn on the Crazy Horse Camping Loop begins with site 25 on the right and continues with spacious sites and large, level tent pads. Site 31 has a great view of the inlet area, where fishing boats drift with the winds searching for that perfect spot. Huge pines shade the entire campground, including site 36, which is a great tent site down a small hill next to a dry creek. Even if you have to drive for a shower, this is rustic tent camping at its best.

Returning to the park road, make a right turn and then an immediate left into Buffalo Hide Campground. This loop road has 24 sites, all with lake views. Proceed to sites 9, 10, 12, 14, and 16 for premier waterfront properties sheltered by huge pine trees. They offer excellent vantage points for observing the local wildlife, including, perhaps, a brief glimpse of the exotic red-plumed male pileated woodpecker.

As a final stop on the main road, a left turn takes you to the boat ramp for unlimited fishing opportunities along 1,200 miles of shoreline. Continue straight ahead to the Arrowhead

A solitary table under the towering pines is the place to be, anytime of year.

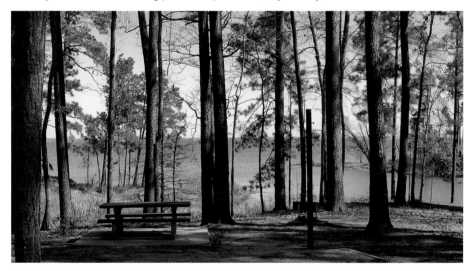

KEY INFORMATION

ADDRESS: Indian Mounds Campground, Forest Service Road 130, Burkeville, TX 75932

OPERATED BY: Sabine River Authority of Texas

CONTACT: 409-565-2273, tinyurl.com/tbindianmounds; no reservations accepted

OPEN: Year-round

SITES: 35

EACH SITE: Picnic table, lantern hook, fire ring, central water

ASSIGNMENT: First come, first served

REGISTRATION: At self-pay station

FACILITIES: Boat ramp, portable toilets

PARKING: At each site

FEE: $4

ELEVATION: 232'

RESTRICTIONS:
PETS: On leash only

FIRES: In fire rings only

ALCOHOL: Prohibited

VEHICLES: 2/site

OTHER: Maximum 8 people/site; guests must leave by 10 p.m.; quiet time 10 p.m.–7 a.m.; bring your own firewood or charcoal; pick up main supplies in Hemphill; gathering firewood prohibited

Camping Loop, where there are no tables, water, or restrooms. However, it doesn't matter, because these primitive campsites are located on an elevated peninsula providing spectacular 180-degree views of the massive reservoir and the state of Louisiana on the far shore.

After choosing your site, head to the 185,000-acre reservoir for one of Texas's premier fishing locations. A boat will allow access to countless coves and inlets where you can fish, bird-watch, or just float with the breeze.

If hiking is your main interest, return to Indian Mounds Wilderness Area on FM 3382 or to Lake View Campground 16 miles southeast of Hemphill via TX 87 and Forest Service Road 105. This small campground has 10 tent sites and is at the trailhead for the Trail Between the Lakes. This 28-mile hiking trail extends from Lakeview Campground to US 96 within sight of the easternmost point of Sam Rayburn Reservoir. The trail is the result of cooperation between the Sierra Club and the U.S. Forest Service, and it passes through Moore Plantation Wildlife Management Area and several colonies of red-cockaded woodpeckers. Be sure to check with the local forest service office for information about camping restrictions in these areas, especially during hunting season. The trail is open to hikers only, so your wilderness experience should be excellent. Bring your binoculars and fishing gear to this easternmost park for a great tent-camping experience.

VOICES FROM THE CAMPFIRE AND RECOMMENDED READING

A stationary camp is quickly cluttered up. Stay too long or return to the same camping place too often, and the inevitable encrustation appears. You fix up a cupboard, install a bench between two trees, improvise a table. These and other little conveniences may be nothing more than a few pimples, but they indicate that the disease of civilization is setting in.
Roy Bedichek, *Adventures with a Texas Naturalist* (Garden City, NY, Doubleday, 1947).

The woods were full of peril—rattlesnakes and water moccasins and nests of copperheads; bobcats, bears, coyotes, wolves, and wild boar; loony hillbillies destabilized by gross quantities of impure corn liquor and generations of profoundly unbiblical sex; rabies-crazed skunks, raccoons, and squirrels; . . . poison ivy, poison sumac, poison oak, and poison salamanders; even a scattering of moose lethally deranged by a parasitic worm that burrows a nest in their brains and befuddles them into chasing hapless hikers through remote, sunny meadows and into glacial lakes.

Bill Bryson, *A Walk in the Woods* (New York, Broadway Books, 1998).

BACKCOUNTRY ADVENTURES

While the reservoir is an obvious boating destination, the 54-mile section of the Sabine River below the dam is one of the more scenic, high-quality, and remote waterways in the state. Only one bridge crosses over the river, and a true feeling of wilderness is possible. The put-in is just below the dam, and the takeout is at the TX 63 crossing. Don't miss it or you will be forced to endure another 40 miles of solitude until you reach US 190.

BEST LOCAL FOOD AND DRINK

Because this long, narrow, and remote reservoir forms a portion of the Texas/Louisiana border, the food choices are not limited to the Texas side. Check out Fisherman's Galley (318-256-0757) and Country Boy Restaurant (318-256-3953) in Many, Louisiana, or the Feed Store Cafe (409-787-3335) in Hemphill, Texas.

Toledo Bend Reservoir: Indian Mounds Campground

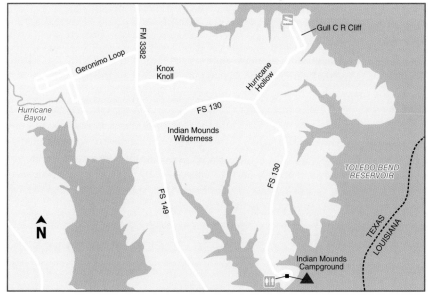

GETTING THERE

From Hemphill, take FM 83 for 7 miles east. Turn right onto FM 3382 and drive 3.9 miles. Turn left into Indian Mounds Recreation Area (Forest Service Road 130).

GPS COORDINATES: N31° 18.864' W93° 41.850'

43

⛺ Toledo Bend Reservoir:

RAGTOWN RECREATION AREA

Beauty: ★★★★ / Privacy: ★★★ / Spaciousness: ★★★ / Quiet: ★★★ / Security: ★★★ / Cleanliness: ★★★

Ragtown is not your typical lake campground.

As you leave the fast-growing city of Lufkin, the creature comforts of fast food and modern mall life disappear in a hurry. They are replaced by the tall pines, flowering redbuds, and dogwoods as you move into a part of Deep East Texas visited only by locals and the lucky tent camper searching for that perfect outdoor experience. Your quest takes you across the Angelina River, through the Angelina National Forest, and into the Sabine River Basin.

At the town of Milam, a left turn on TX 87 takes you toward Ragtown Recreation Area. As you head north on 87, this scenic road roughly parallels the massive reservoir hidden to the east. Approaching Ragtown Recreation Area, you find very quickly this is not the typical lake campground, but a rugged piece of territory marked by massive pine trees and steep ravines. It is a reminder of the difference between a tree farm and a forest with a mix of pines, hardwoods, and understory plants. There is even an area for the critically endangered red-cockaded woodpecker. The 20-year legal fight over this bird helped save much of the national forest from clear-cutting.

After paying at the self-registration station, you enter Ragtown on the narrow road that leads down the hill to the water's edge and boat ramp to the right. Stay straight for the camping area and the camp-host site on your right, along with site 1, which backs up to a heavily wooded ravine, has a nice view of the water, and is across the street from one of the only water sources. Just up the hill are the modern restrooms and showers on the left.

A quiet visit during the week is a reward in itself.

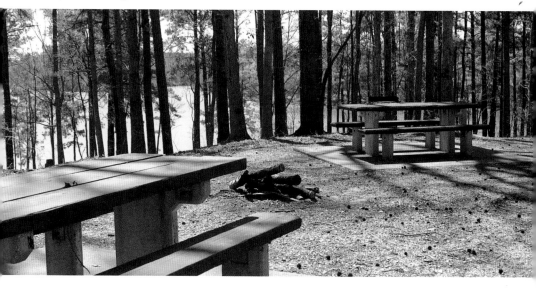

KEY INFORMATION

ADDRESS: Ragtown Recreational Area, Forest Service Road 132, Shelbyville, TX 75932

OPERATED BY: Sabine River Authority of Texas

CONTACT: 409-565-2273, tinyurl.com /tbindianmounds; no reservations accepted

OPEN: Year-round

SITES: 25

EACH SITE: Picnic table, upright fire grate or ring, lantern hook

ASSIGNMENT: First come, first served

REGISTRATION: At self-pay station

FACILITIES: Modern restrooms and showers, boat ramp

PARKING: At each site

FEE: Single site, $5; double site, $8

ELEVATION: 305'

RESTRICTIONS:

PETS: On leash only

FIRES: In fire grates or rings only

ALCOHOL: Prohibited

VEHICLES: 2/site

OTHER: Maximum 8 people/site; guests must leave by 10 p.m.; quiet time 10 p.m.–6 a.m.; bring firewood or charcoal; pick up main supplies in Center, Logansport, or Hemphill; gathering firewood prohibited

Continue up the hill for more heavily treed sites, including a number of double sites. At the top of the hill are some of the premier tent sites in Texas. On the left side, just after more modern restrooms, look for sites 11–14, 16, 19, 21, and 22 for spectacular views out over the Toledo Bend Reservoir. These elevated sites also allow for some breeze and a little relief from the hot weather of summer. At road's end, there is a small circle drive and an unnumbered spot (probably 25), which puts your tent out on a small peninsula for 180-degree views. The site is level with the water's edge, which is only a short walk down the hill.

Considering the easy access to Mother Nature's Trail, the lack of electricity or water at every site is really no problem to the tent camper looking for a perfect Deep East Texas destination. One-mile Mother Nature's Trail loops around the campground and provides great views of the north end of Toledo Bend Reservoir's 185,000 surface acres and its 65 miles of open water. After you pick your tent site, return to the bottom of the hill and head to the water. The world-class fishing includes black bass and crappie. There are also numerous photography options, including sunrise shots over the lake and bird-watching of all types. In addition to the endangered red-cockaded woodpecker, the area includes bald eagles, ospreys, cranes, herons, hawks, owls, and even a few loons and pelicans on the southern end of the reservoir. Fall is especially beautiful, as the mix of oak, maple, sycamore, cypress, and hickory trees provide bright yellows and deep reds in contrast with the towering pines.

As you leave the campground, take time to visit the small communities of Milam and Geneva, which were stops on the El Camino Real, Texas's oldest trail and highway. The El Camino Real was first used by the Caddo Indians, then by French and Spanish explorers, and finally by a flood of new Texans, including Stephen F. Austin.

VOICES FROM THE CAMPFIRE AND RECOMMENDED READING

Any fool can destroy trees. They cannot run away; and if they could, they would still be destroyed,—chased and hunted down as long as fun or a dollar could be got out of their bark hides, branching horns, or magnificent bole backbones. . . . God has cared for these trees, saved them from drought, disease, avalanches, and a thousand straining, leveling tempests and floods; but he cannot save them from fools,—only Uncle Sam can do that.

John Muir, "The American Forests," *The Atlantic,* August, 1897.

BACKCOUNTRY ADVENTURES

Pick up a detailed map from the Sabine River Authority of Texas (sratx.org) and head out on this 185,000-acre body of water, which stretches about 65 miles from the dam to Logansport. You can explore any number of areas with inviting names ranging from Sunshine Bay to Rebel Ridge Cove to Cow Bayou. Bring plenty of supplies for a full day of exploring.

BEST LOCAL FOOD AND DRINK

In Milam, especially good options at Martin's Corner (409-625-3000) include breakfast and fish. In Hemphill to the south, stop by Hemphill BBQ (409-787-1814), especially for brisket and ribs, or the Feed Store Cafe (409-787-3335) for meals described as upscale and fresh.

Toledo Bend Reservoir: Ragtown Recreation Area

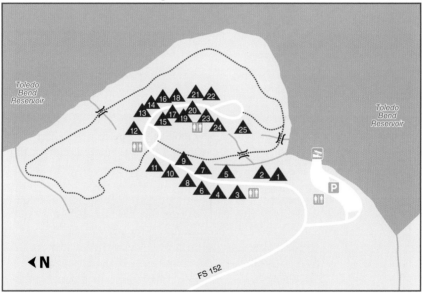

GETTING THERE

From Lufkin, drive 56 miles east on TX 103 to Milam. Turn left onto TX 87 and drive north 23 miles. Turn right onto FM 139 to FM 3184. Ragtown is 4 miles ahead.

GPS COORDINATES: N31° 40.968' W93° 49.650'

NORTHEAST TEXAS AND CADDO LAKE AREA

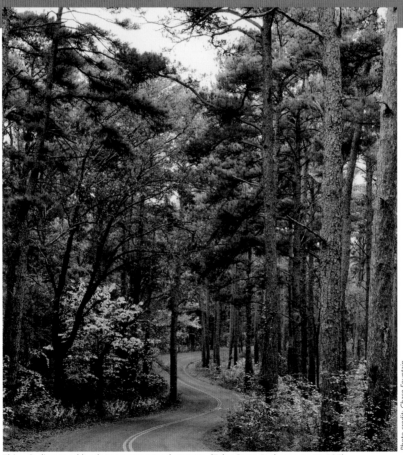

Photo credit: *Chase Fountain*

This winding road leads to your next adventure. (Tyler State Park; see page 185)

44

⛺ Atlanta State Park

Beauty: ★★★ / Privacy: ★★ / Spaciousness: ★★ / Quiet: ★★ / Security: ★★★ / Cleanliness: ★★★

As you pick your tent site, watch the sky for large soaring red-tailed hawks.

Once the home of the Caddo Indians, this 1,475-acre remote park is known as "Nature's best-kept secret in Northeast Texas." Just a few miles from the town of Atlanta, Texas, and the Arkansas border, the entrance road is bordered by thick stands of pines and oaks, which make perfect shelter for the three major campgrounds. Passing the headquarters, the cool breezes of fall and the trees beginning to change promise a rewarding camping experience as you turn left toward the Knights Bluff camping area on your right. Make another immediate right for sites 1–8, which have water and electricity. These well-spaced sites have an occasional RV, but RV campers usually go toward sites 10–23 with full hookups and even a satellite dish or two.

Continue toward the lake for a large picnic area overlooking the massive 20,300-acre Wright Patman Lake. This reservoir was built by the U.S. Army Corps of Engineers and supports a wide variety of water sports, including fishing for crappie, catfish, sand bass, and black bass. It also serves as a stopover for large flocks of migrating birds heading south for the winter.

Returning to the main road, travel past the turn toward the park entrance, continuing toward the Wilkins Creek camping area. Note the Hickory Hollow Nature Trail on your

This wilderness lake is far from the big city.

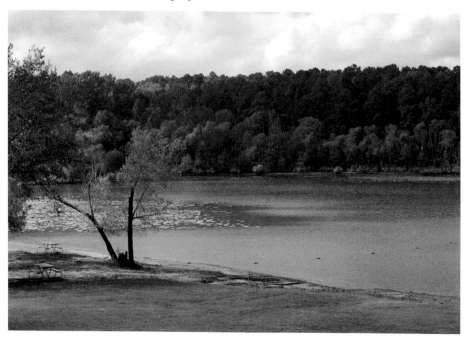

KEY INFORMATION

ADDRESS: 927 Park Road 42, Atlanta, TX 75551

CONTACT: 903-796-6476, tpwd.texas.gov/state-parks/atlanta

OPERATED BY: Texas Parks & Wildlife Department

OPEN: Year-round

SITES: 58 (in three campground areas)

EACH SITE: Picnic table, fire ring, electrical hookup, water, tent pad

ASSIGNMENT: First come, first served until site-specific reservation system begins in 2018

REGISTRATION: At park office or reserve at texas.reserveworld.com or 512-389-8900

FACILITIES: Modern restrooms

PARKING: At each site

FEE: $14–$16, $3/person entrance fee

ELEVATION: 246'

RESTRICTIONS:

PETS: On leash only

FIRES: Fire rings or upright grills only

ALCOHOL: Prohibited in all public/ outdoor areas

VEHICLES: 2/site

OTHER: Maximum 8 people/site; quiet time 10 p.m.–6 a.m.; canoes for rent; fishing tackle to loan; bring your own firewood or charcoal; park store has T-shirts, hats, fishing supplies; pick up main supplies in Atlanta or Queen City; gathering firewood prohibited

right. This trail is part of a 3-mile system into the backcountry and eventually connects to the White Oak Ridge camping area.

As you pass the trailhead parking lot, turn right into the Wilkins Creek camping area. These sites have water and electricity, with terrain ideal for tents. Sites 24–33 are nicely wooded, but look for sites 32, 34, and 36 for good tent pads constructed along a ridgeline and backing up to a heavily treed and rugged ravine. As you pick your tent site, listen and watch the sky for high soaring red-tailed hawks, whose screams might sound like expressions of pure enjoyment but really indicate that they're defending their territory.

Returning to the main road, turn right and travel 0.1 mile, then make another right into White Oak Ridge camping area. The bathrooms and showers are on your left and the winding road with steep inclines makes it less desirable for large RVs. The sites sit on a ridgeline that stretches toward the lake. Sites 52–55 give you elevated lake views and a little extra breeze during hot weather. There are level tent pads and a sense of remoteness, as long as the weekend crowds have returned to their RV areas and leave this little-known piece of Northeast Texas beauty to you and your tent.

VOICES FROM THE CAMPFIRE AND RECOMMENDED READING

I suppose each of us has his own fantasy of how he wants to die. I would like to go out in a blaze of glory, myself, or maybe simply disappear someday, far out in the heart of the wilderness I love, all by myself, alone with the Universe and whatever God may happen to be looking on. Disappear—and never return.

Author's note: Edward Abbey in a letter to his father, Paul Revere Abbey, March 14, 1975)

Edward Abbey, Postcards from Ed (Minneapolis, Milkweed Editions, 2006)

BACKCOUNTRY ADVENTURES

This jewel of an area offers many options for enjoying the outdoors. Bring your fishing pole to catch some catfish or crappie. A pair of binoculars will help you spot many rare and beautiful birds, especially during migration in early spring and early fall. Rent a canoe or bring a canoe or kayak to explore the coves when the winds are calm.

BEST LOCAL FOOD AND DRINK

If you're not in the mood to cook out at your campsite, stop in Atlanta at Luigi's Italian Cafe (903-796-7020; luigisitaliancafe.us) or the Rabbit Patch (903-650-9602). For good barbecue, visit Rickey's Rib Shack (706 Loop 59, Atlanta) or Tommy's (903-796-5719). For some Cajun flavor, try Roux-Ga-Roux Seafood (430-562-7123).

Atlanta State Park

GETTING THERE

From Atlanta, travel 2 miles north on US 59. Exit onto FM 96 and go west 9 miles. Turn right onto FM 1154 and travel north 2 miles to the Park Road 42 entrance. (FM 1154 dead-ends at the park.)

From the intersection of I-369 and US 59 in Texarkana, take US 59 S for 15.6 miles. Turn right onto County Road 3541 and drive 1.1 miles. Turn right onto CR 3542 and drive just 0.2 mile, then turn left onto CR 3543 and drive 0.6 mile. Turn right onto FM 96 and drive 5.0 miles. Turn right onto FM 1154 and drive 1.7 miles. Turn left onto Park Road 42 and drive to the park entrance.

GPS COORDINATES: N33° 13.833' W94° 14.983'

45

Bonham State Park

Beauty: ★★★ / Privacy: ★★ / Spaciousness: ★★ / Quiet: ★★ / Security: ★★★ / Cleanliness: ★★★★

Visit the lakeside pavilion here for a possible glimpse of resident Canadian snow geese enjoying the breeze and open water.

As you travel northeast from the traffic jams of Dallas and its booming suburbs, the rolling countryside of TX 121 is a welcome relief. The trees begin to outnumber the cars, and the spaciousness of rural Texas allows you to relax your grip on the steering wheel. From the small entrance station at Bonham, you will proceed into a canopy of huge trees shading the road. At 0.4 mile, you cross the Lake Loop Trail, so be sure to watch for mountain bikers. At 0.7 mile, you'll spot a group tent-camping area on the right with multiple picnic tables, upright grills, and central water.

At the intersection, turn left and the tent-only sites are on your immediate left. Starting with site 21, this small campground has a nice view of the lake. Site 20 is set back into the trees for extra privacy. Sites 15–19 are also in the trees but are located a little closer to RV sites 1–14. These RV sites have electricity hookups if your tent-camping group needs a little modern comfort. The relatively new restrooms and showers (even heated) are a short walk up the road on the right, and park headquarters is on the left in a stone building built by the Civilian Conservation Corps in the 1930s. It has not only a commanding view of the lake but also a large covered pavilion perfect for family reunions or other large groups. This pavilion also sits lakeside with easy access to the fishing pier and provides an ideal view of the resident Canadian snow geese enjoying the breeze and open water.

CCC stonework is a marvel of hard work and rustic beauty.

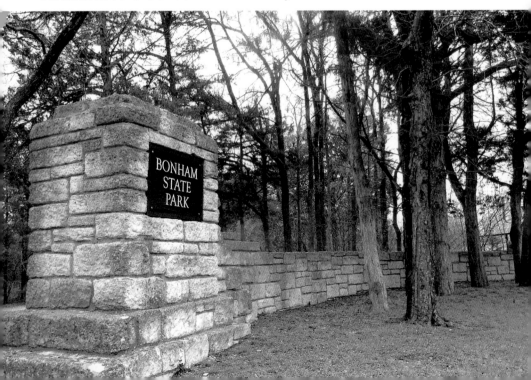

KEY INFORMATION

ADDRESS: 1363 State Park Road 24, Bonham, TX 75418

CONTACT: 903-583-5022, tpwd.texas.gov/state-parks/bonham

OPERATED BY: Texas Parks & Wildlife Department

OPEN: Year-round

SITES: 7, one group camping area (50 person max)

EACH SITE: Picnic tables, upright grills, fire rings, lantern hooks, and central water

ASSIGNMENT: First come, first served until site-specific reservation system begins in 2018

REGISTRATION: At headquarters or reserve at texas.reserveworld.com or 512-389-8900

FACILITIES: Modern restrooms and showers across from park headquarters

PARKING: At each site

FEE: $15/night, group area $75/night; $4/person entrance fee

ELEVATION: 630'

RESTRICTIONS:

PETS: On leash only

FIRES: In fire rings or upright grills only

ALCOHOL: Prohibited in all public/outdoor areas

VEHICLES: 2/site

OTHER: Maximum 8 people/site; guests must leave by 10 p.m.; quiet time 10 p.m.–6 a.m.; bring your own firewood or charcoal; pick up main supplies in Bonham; gathering firewood prohibited

---

After setting up your tent, get your hiking boots on or tune up the mountain bike for miles of trails, which disappear into the heavy woods. These bike trails offer moderate difficulty and require helmets for safety. You should also carry plenty of water for proper hydration in the Texas heat. Luckily, the park contains mature stands of Shumard oaks, green ashes, cottonwoods, and mighty oaks to provide shade for hikers and bikers.

After working hard on the trails, head for the small but scenic 65-acre lake, which has a swimming area and canoe and paddleboat rentals. The lake provides a tranquil background for a relaxing afternoon with a good book or fishing off the pier.

As you leave this central area, cross the one-lane bridge for a 0.4-mile scenic return drive to the entrance station. Follow signs back to Bonham for a taste of Texas hospitality, and be sure to visit the Sam Rayburn Library. This Texas legend held power in Washington with the likes of LBJ and FDR.

VOICES FROM THE CAMPFIRE AND RECOMMENDED READING

I decided then and there that real environmental change had to begin with us—you and me. We can't wait for our leaders. We don't have time. These days we worry about growing terrorist activities, but other problems that could sicken and kill whole generations of our children and grandchildren are environmental ones—water degradation, topsoil loss, air pollution, and climate change. Some of today's youth may feel they have inherited problems too great to do anything about. They have not. All it takes is getting involved.

Richard M. Donovan, *Paddling the Wild Neches* (College Station, Texas A&M University Press, 2006).

I also recommend picking up *Encounters with the Archdruid* by John McPhee (Farrar, Straus and Giroux, 1971), which includes narratives about a conservationist and three of his natural enemies.

BACKCOUNTRY ADVENTURES

While the canoe and paddleboat rentals will help relax your big-city nerves, the 8.8 miles of trails offer both main routes and enough auxiliary trails to keep your ride interesting and challenging. The group area can hold up to 50 of your closest friends and is surrounded by some nice tree cover and enough picnic tables to hold your group meals. Get to the site early and pitch your tent toward the back for extra shade and privacy. The park staff is very friendly.

BEST LOCAL FOOD AND DRINK

The city of Bonham is a thriving Northeast Texas community with plenty of food choices. Try Muddbones (903-583-5385) for best burger, Roma (903-583-3292; romabonham.com) for Italian, Bamboo House (903-583-6969) for top-notch Asian foods, The Breakfast Stop (903-583-2618; bonhambreakfaststop.com) for eggs and cinnamon rolls, Hickory Bar-B-Que (903-583-3081), or Lil's Chuckwagon (903-583-9247).

Bonham State Park

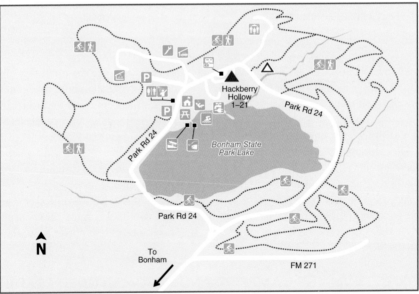

GETTING THERE

From the intersection of I-635 and US 75 in Dallas, take US 75 N for 25.6 miles. Take Exit 44 for TX 121 N/Bonham and drive 29.2 miles. Turn right onto FM 1629 and drive 2.9 miles. Turn left onto TX 78 N and drive 0.9 mile. Turn right onto FM 271 and drive 1.9 miles. Turn left onto Park Road 24 and keep left for the park entrance.

GPS COORDINATES: N33° 33.586' W96° 9.018'

46

Caddo Lake State Park

Beauty: ★★★★ / Privacy: ★★★ / Spaciousness: ★★★ / Quiet: ★★★ / Security: ★★★ / Cleanliness: ★★★

Caddo Lake offers large sites with lake views enhanced by hanging moss and huge cypress trees.

Named after the Caddo Indians, this natural wonderland has been inhabited for at least 12,000 years and continues as one of the premier wetland parks in the world. In 1993, this largest natural lake in Texas was designated a Wetland of International Importance under the Ramsar Convention. Originally formed by a natural logjam, this maze of slow-moving bayous and backwaters covers more than 25,000 acres and provides an ideal setting for tent camping and low-speed water sports.

As you pass the park entrance, the magic of this place appears almost immediately in the form of thick forests of pine, oak, and hickory draped with Spanish moss. Following the main park road for about 1.5 miles, you descend a steep hill and then turn left at the T-intersection toward the camping areas. At the central parking area, stay to your right and cross the wooden bridge into Mill Pond Camping Area for one of Texas's best tent-camping areas. With the lake at your back door, sites 65, 64, and 63 are to your immediate right. These large sites have views of the lake that are only enhanced by the hanging moss and huge cypress trees growing in the shallow water. Proceeding farther, sites 62–57 are at the turnaround point and provide the most privacy and solitude. The remaining sites are a little closer together, but the setting has such beauty that even some togetherness is no real distraction, especially on a moonlit walk to the fishing pier just off the central parking area. If the hanging moss and swamp flowers don't give you a feeling of wilderness, then just remember there are alligators in the area, along with 70 species of fish.

Just being in this wilderness water park is soothing to any overworked city dweller.

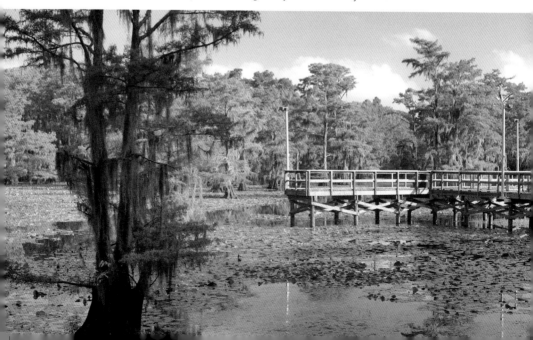

KEY INFORMATION

ADDRESS: 245 Park Road 2,
Karnack, TX 75661

CONTACT: 903-679-3351,
tpwd.texas.gov/state-parks/caddo-lake

OPERATED BY: Texas Parks & Wildlife
Department

OPEN: Year-round

SITES: 20

EACH SITE: Water, fire ring, picnic table,
lantern hook

ASSIGNMENT: First come, first served
until site-specific reservation system
begins in 2018

REGISTRATION: At headquarters or reserve at
texas.reserveworld.com or 512-389-8900

FACILITIES: Restrooms and showers, canoe
rentals, park store, recreation hall

PARKING: At each site

FEES: Tent camping $10/night at Mill Pond;
$4/person entrance fee

ELEVATION: 275'

RESTRICTIONS:

PETS: On leash only

FIRES: In fire rings

ALCOHOL: Prohibited in all public/
outdoor areas

VEHICLES: 2/site

OTHER: Maximum 8 people/site; guests must
leave by 10 p.m.; quiet time 10 p.m.–6 a.m.;
bring your own firewood or charcoal; limited
supplies at concession store at Saw Mill
Pond; main supplies in Marshall or Jefferson;
gathering firewood prohibited

As you leave Mill Pond, the park store is on your left. There you can rent canoes or buy souvenirs, but no food or drinks are available. (There is no longer an on-site concessionaire offering boat tours.) The restrooms and showers are on your right near the entrance to the RV areas and the one-way exit road. Follow this road 0.2 mile up the hill and make a left toward the boat ramp. Look for the Caddo Forest Trail on your right, which is listed as a 0.75-mile nature walk but connects to a series of steep hikes and eventually to the old Civilian Conservation Corps Pavilion. The trail also ends in a parking and picnic area with great views of the Big Cypress Bayou. Following the one-way road returns you to the central parking area for Mill Pond and the concession store.

Be sure to give yourself a little extra time at Caddo to soak up the natural beauty and rich history. After the Caddo Indians, the area became a sort of hideout for renegades and misfits whose contempt for the law (especially during Prohibition) remains a local tradition. The lake was also a stop on the steamboat route from New Orleans to Jefferson, which explains how this transplanted piece of French architecture landed deep in the Texas piney woods.

VOICES FROM THE CAMPFIRE AND RECOMMENDED READING

We can never have enough of nature. We must be refreshed by the sight of inexhaustible vigor, vast and titanic features, the sea-coast with its wrecks, the wilderness with its living and its decaying trees, the thunder-cloud, and the rain which lasts three weeks and produces freshets. We need to witness our own limits transgressed, and some life pasturing freely where we never wander.

Henry David Thoreau, *Walden, or Life in the Woods* (Boston, Ticknor and Fields, 1854).

Also check out *In Wildness Is the Preservation of the World* by Henry David Thoreau, with photographs by Eliot Porter and an introduction by David Brower (Sierra Club Books, 1962).

BACKCOUNTRY ADVENTURES

Several boat tours are based out of Uncertain. If you are an explorer type, you can rent a kayak or canoe to enter the labyrinth of waterways, which all seem to look alike after you start the return trip. Be sure to bring enough gear to spend the night in your boat should you become lost. Remember that cell service is very spotty in this wilderness area, so don't depend on the digital age to rescue you from this ancient and foreboding landscape.

BEST LOCAL FOOD AND DRINK

This far East Texas park is flanked by the great towns of Karnack and Uncertain. You can get a great meal at Dad's Pizza Pad (903-789-3231) or the Uncertain General Store & Grill (903-789-3292), or go into the historic town of Jefferson and stop in at Kitt's Kornbread Sandwich and Pie Bar (903-665-0505; kittskornbread.com) (with the slogan "This ain't your mama's cornbread!"). If you want a special treat, and you're not too stinky from the trail, enjoy fine dining at the Stillwater Inn (903-665-8415; stillwaterinn.com).

Caddo Lake State Park

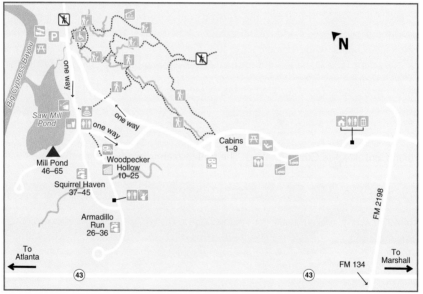

GETTING THERE

In the city of Marshall on US 59, turn right onto TX 43 and drive 14 miles. Turn right onto FM 2198 and go 0.5 mile. Turn left on Park Road 2; park entrance is straight ahead.

GPS COORDINATES: N32° 40.800' W94° 10.602'

47

Caddo National Grasslands

Beauty: ★★★ / Privacy: ★★★ / Spaciousness: ★★★ / Quiet: ★★★ / Security: ★★ / Cleanliness: ★★★

Tall pines mixed with mighty oaks impart a special feeling during the first cool afternoons of fall.

In a state as large as Texas, the hidden gems are exactly that: hidden. This series of three campgrounds is easily overlooked in the 17,873-acre Caddo National Grasslands. While the massive area north of Bonham is clearly marked on state road maps, its very name implies vast, open savannahs with little shade or protection for the tent camper. However, nothing could be further from the truth in this heavily wooded forest containing enough lakes and creeks for a true wilderness experience.

After turning east on FM 409, the first campground is Bois D'Arc Trailhead Overnight Area 2.4 miles on the right. The self-pay station and compost toilets are straight ahead, with the campsite loop starting to the right. This heavily treed campground is the prime meeting place for the local equestrian community, whose horse trailers and Texan friendliness fill the sites on weekends. This area is the starting point for five different trail loops totaling 28 miles through the rugged Caddo Wildlife Management Area. You might encounter red and gray fox, gulls, quail, white-tailed deer, wild turkey, and two-legged deer hunters in season, so be alert. Site 15 is at the far end of the 0.6-mile loop and offers extra space and privacy but a long walk to the toilet.

Returning to FM 409, turn right for 1.7 miles and then right into Coffee Mill Lake Recreation Area. This campground offers lake views from every site, and all sites are nicely spaced. There is a boat ramp, and the large trees give plenty of welcome shade. Sites 12 and

This small tent campground has just the right feel.

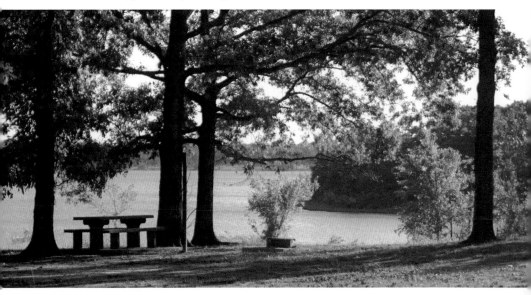

KEY INFORMATION

ADDRESS: FM 409, Telephone, TX 75488

CONTACT: 940-627-5475, tinyurl.com/ lbjnatlgrass; no reservations accepted

OPERATED BY: U.S. Forest Service

OPEN: Year-round

SITES: 24, 1 group site in Bois D'Arc, 13 in Coffee Mill Lake, 11 in West Lake Crockett

EACH SITE: Picnic table, fire ring, lantern hook, central water

ASSIGNMENT: First come, first served

REGISTRATION: Self-pay stations

FACILITIES: Composting toilets

PARKING: At each site

FEE: $4–$6/night

ELEVATION: 499'

RESTRICTIONS:

PETS: On leash only; 14-day maximum stay

FIRES: In fire rings only

ALCOHOL: Prohibited

VEHICLES: 2/site

OTHER: Maximum 7 people/site; guests must leave by 10 p.m.; quiet time 10 p.m.–6 a.m.; bring your own firewood or charcoal; pick up main supplies in Bonham; gathering firewood allowed only if down and dead

13 are close enough to be called lakefront, but there are no bad places in this small park to put your tent and do a little fishing or just relaxing.

Returning to FM 409, turn right, travel 3 miles, and turn right again into the West Lake Crockett Campground, which is surrounded on three sides by water. This small, 10-site campground is perfectly placed to get the lake breeze and unparalleled views at sunrise or sunset. The tall pines mixed with the mighty oaks impart a special feeling during the first cool afternoons of fall, when the leaves are turning and beginning to cover the ground. The summer crowds have gone home and you are left to enjoy a moment of solitude in this little-known corner of Northeast Texas.

After you select your site, head out on Bois D'Arc Trail for some wilderness hiking or a cross-country equestrian adventure. The topography is moderately strenuous, so bring sufficient food and water to be out all day. You should also check with the local U.S. Forest Service office to find out if any areas are open during hunting season or if specific trails cross some of the remaining patchwork of private property. As you enjoy this great trail system, look for some really nice natural areas near Coffee Mill Creek, which eventually ends in Coffee Mill Lake.

Returning to the Bois D'Arc trailhead, take your fishing gear over to Coffee Mill Lake or West Lake Crockett for some peace and quiet. These small campgrounds are the perfect locations to throw in a line and read a good book. Add in a small fire and you have a great escape from the big city.

VOICES FROM THE CAMPFIRE AND RECOMMENDED READING

These fires at night brought cheer and fellowship. We would talk of the happenings of the day and of the plans for tomorrow; of the perplexing problems of school and of home. . . . As the sparks rose to the tops of the trees and disappeared into the firmament, we would dream dreams that only boys can dream.

William O. Douglas, Chapter X: The Campfire, *Of Men and Mountains* (New York, Harper & Brothers, 1950).

BACKCOUNTRY ADVENTURES

With 28 miles of trail loops, you can take your horse or hiking boots on any number of adventures. If the equestrian crowd is in camp, make new friends and find out what trails they are using, so you can hike the others for smoother footing. Or be a true Texan and learn to ride these very powerful animals.

BEST LOCAL FOOD AND DRINK

With the park located just north of Bonham, try Muddbones (903-583-5385) for best burger, Roma (903-583-3292; romabonham.com) for Italian, Bamboo House (903-583-6969) for top-notch Asian fare, The Breakfast Stop (903-583-2618; bonhambreakfaststop .com), Hickory Bar-B-Que (903-583-3081), or Lil's Chuckwagon (903-583-9247).

Caddo National Grasslands

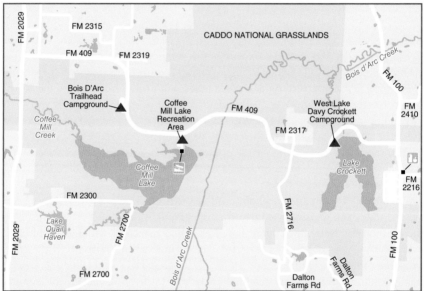

GETTING THERE

From Telephone, take FM 2029 south 1 mile to FM 409 and turn left. Bois D'Arc is on the right. From Bonham, drive north 6 miles on TX 78 and turn right onto FM 1396. Drive 9 miles and turn left onto FM 2029. After 3.9 miles, turn right onto FM 409. Bois D'Arc is on the right.

See the profile for directions to Coffee Mill Lake and West Lake Crockett Campgrounds.

GPS COORDINATES: N33° 44.184' W95° 58.398'

Cooper Lake State Park:
SOUTH SULPHUR UNIT

Beauty: ★★★★ / Privacy: ★★★★ / Spaciousness: ★★★★ / Quiet: ★★★★ / Security: ★★★ / Cleanliness: ★★★

Each site has its own private trail and feels more like a backpacking experience.

Another hidden gem in the Texas State Park system lies off the beaten tourist path, but avid tent campers should not miss it. Located on the south shore of Cooper Lake, the South Sulphur Unit offers the usual park activities, but the huge, 19,300-acre lake and more than 25 miles of shoreline give a wilderness feel to all visitors, but especially the tent camper.

After leaving the entrance station, the park road winds through thick stands of oak trees and rolling hills. With each mile, the terrain gets a little wilder until you pass the Buggy Whip Equestrian Camping Area 2.3 miles on your left and enter the Deer Haven RV area. Just as you pass the restrooms and showers on your left, watch for the sign on your right for Oak Grove Camping Area. After parking in the paved central parking area, grab your gear and follow the easy trail to some of the best tent camping around.

Beginning with site number 88 on your far right, each site has its own private trail and feels more like a backpacking experience. Sites 92, 94–99, and 101 and 102 are waterfront property where you can hear the waves while lying in your sleeping bag. Most of the sites are divided by heavy brush for extra privacy. At the end of the trail, sites 99 and 101 even share their own beach. The entire campground is arranged on a peninsula, so you are separate from the RV areas and also have great views of sunrise or sunset, depending on your final site selection. There are no bathrooms in the Oak Grove campground, but enough nature to wander into as necessary with the restrooms and showers less than 5 minutes away by car.

These sites provide great water views without leaving your tent.

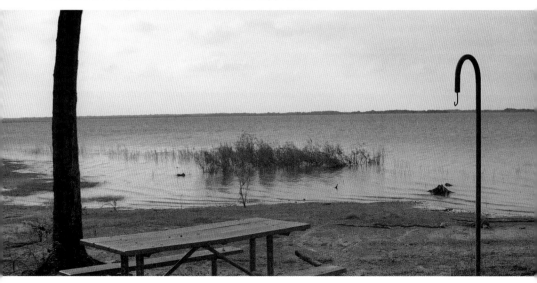

KEY INFORMATION

ADDRESS: 1690 FM 3505, Sulphur Springs, TX 75482

CONTACT: 903-945-5256, tpwd.texas.gov/state-parks/cooper-lake

OPERATED BY: Texas Parks & Wildlife Department

OPEN: Year-round

SITES: 15

EACH SITE: Fire ring, picnic table, lantern hook, water nearby

ASSIGNMENT: First come, first served until site-specific reservation system begins in 2018

REGISTRATION: At headquarters or reserve at texas.reserveworld.com or 512-389-8900

FACILITIES: Modern restrooms and showers on main road

PARKING: Central parking

FEE: $10, $5/person entrance fee

ELEVATION: 472'

RESTRICTIONS:

PETS: On leash only

FIRES: In fire rings only

ALCOHOL: Prohibited in all public/outdoor areas

VEHICLES: 2/site

OTHER: Maximum 8 people/site; guests must leave by 10 p.m.; quiet time 10 p.m.–6 a.m.; bring your own firewood or charcoal; pick up main supplies in Sulphur Springs; gathering firewood prohibited

As you leave the Oak Grove Area, check out the Buggy Whip Equestrian Area and its 11-mile trail. Returning toward the entrance station, a left turn into the Heron Harbor Day Use Area will bring you to a protected swimming area and the 5-mile Coyote Run Hiking Trail.

A little more than an hour and a half from Dallas, this park is a must-visit for anyone needing a weekend escape. After setting up your tent, go explore this 2,560-acre park surrounding a water reservoir with a wildlife management area. The terrain is rolling and covered with oaks, elms, hackberries, and evergreen eastern red cedars. Hiking and equestrian trails also cross areas of prairie, which are reminders that this portion of Texas still retains a few patches of the great expanses of grassland that run from Texas to the northern plains.

Returning to the main road, travel to Honey Creek Day Use Area or Heron Harbor Day Use Area for some of Texas's best fishing. When the reservoir was created in 1986 by damming the South Sulphur River, a large number of trees were left as habitat for largemouth and white bass, along with catfish and crappie. If you need some exercise, check out the 5-mile Coyote Run Trail. This moderately strenuous hiking trail starts and ends in the Heron Harbor parking lot, which is conveniently located next to the swimming area.

Whether on the trail or in the Oak Grove Camping Area, keep watch for the usual white-tailed deer, armadillos, and raccoons, in addition to the occasional bald eagle or wild turkey. There is also Doctor's Creek Unit on the north side of the lake, but the camping there is primarily for RVs. The area does have additional hiking and biking trails for exploring this 466-acre unit of Cooper Lake State Park.

VOICES FROM THE CAMPFIRE AND RECOMMENDED READING

For a city person, the pace of life out here can take some getting used to.... The journey we're on this morning is referred to as "forest bathing," meaning a slow, watchful walk whose benefits are

said to range from clarity of mind to lowered blood pressure. "It's an active form of meditation,"
says [Hope] Parks, a way to "focus on our senses and how nature awakens them."
  Elaine Glusac, "The Woodland Cure," *American Way,* December, 2016.

BACKCOUNTRY ADVENTURES

The 11-mile equestrian trail and the 5-mile hiking trail will give you great opportunities to look for bald eagles, which have made parts of Northeast Texas their year-round home. Look for nesting sites in tall trees or even cross-country power lines, whose towers seem ideal for supporting the nest. Returning to the water, the fishing is a prime attraction and the protected swimming area is an ideal way to cool down when the Texas heat arrives for the summer.

BEST LOCAL FOOD AND DRINK

Some favorites in the small town of Cooper include Tejano's Tex-Mex (903-300-3315) and Fatboy's BBQ (903-300-3287) and twisty fries. For a great breakfast served all day, check out Little Chef (903-300-3800) in Cooper or Pioneer Cafe (903-885-7773) (family style) in Sulphur Springs. Or just stroll around the square in Sulphur Springs for many more options.

Cooper Lake State Park: South Sulphur Unit

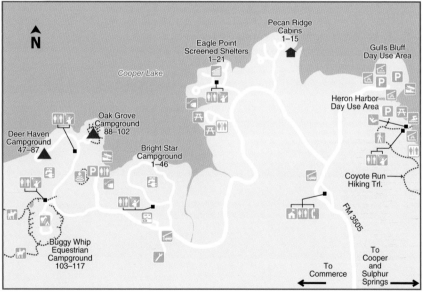

GETTING THERE

From Interstate 30, as it passes through Sulphur Springs, drive north 11.6 miles on TX 19. Turn left onto FM 71 and drive 4.4 miles, then turn right on FM 3505 and drive 1.5 miles to Park Road 8154A.

GPS COORDINATES: N33° 17.286' W95° 39.468'

49

Daingerfield State Park

Beauty: ★★★ / Privacy: ★★ / Spaciousness: ★★★ / Quiet: ★★ / Security: ★★★ / Cleanliness: ★★★

The endangered red-cockaded woodpecker has been known to nest in this area.

Deep in the piney woods of Northeast Texas, it is easy to imagine the local Caddo Indians traveling along pathways used for centuries to trade with the Choctaw, Cherokee, and the newly arrived European explorers. This popular transportation route was known as the Caddo Trace and was also used for stage routes and mail routes. It was also traveled during the Civil War.

Against this historical backdrop, the Civilian Conservation Corps (CCC) built Daingerfield State Park from 1935 to 1938 during the Great Depression, to combat unemployment. The well-worn but durable structures remind us of this difficult period and also leave a legacy of beauty for today's tent campers seeking to get away from the modern economic stresses.

After leaving the headquarters, a left turn at 0.2 mile sends you into rugged wilderness terrain and toward Dogwood Camping Area. These large sites are well spaced with water and electricity. Look for site 17 lakeside on the 80-acre Lake Daingerfield, a no-wake lake where you can now rent canoes, kayaks, paddleboards, paddleboats, and flat-bottom boats. The area is also known for its dogwoods, redbuds, cinnamon ferns, and pine-covered hills, where the endangered red-cockaded woodpecker has been known to nest along with its cousin, the large pileated woodpecker. Just listen on a quiet day; you can hear these two beautiful birds hammering for their meals. Each fall, an outline of brilliant colors shows in full glory around the lake from the surrounding sweet gum, oak, and maple trees.

Returning on the main road, turn right just before the day-use area toward Cedar Ridge Camping Loop. Turn right at 0.4 mile to this elevated campground and more-primitive sites

Admiring the afternoon sunlight reflection off this quiet lake is the best way to end the day.

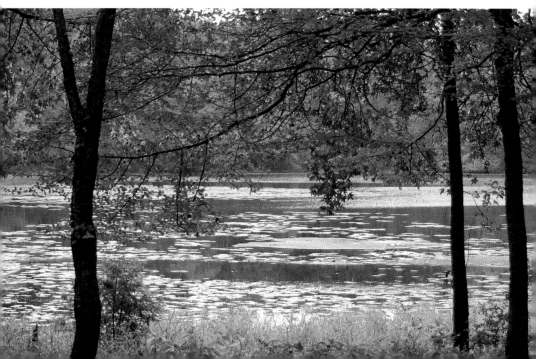

KEY INFORMATION

ADDRESS: 455 Park Road 17, Daingerfield, TX 75638

CONTACT: 903-645-2921, tpwd.texas.gov/state-parks/daingerfield

OPERATED BY: Texas Parks & Wildlife Department

OPEN: Year-round

SITES: 58, including 18 with water only in the Dogwood area

EACH SITE: Central water, picnic table, lantern hook; some have electricity

ASSIGNMENT: First come, first served until site-specific reservation system begins in 2018

REGISTRATION: At headquarters or reserve at texas.reserveworld.com or 512-389-8900

FACILITIES: Modern restrooms and showers at Cedar Ridge/Mountain View, restrooms at Dogwood, interpretive center and park store

PARKING: At each site

FEE: $20–$25 (water and electric), $10 (water only); $4/person entrance fee

ELEVATION: 590'

RESTRICTIONS:

PETS: On leash only

FIRES: In fire rings and grates only

ALCOHOL: Prohibited in all public/outdoor areas

VEHICLES: 2/site

OTHER: Maximum 8 people/site; guests must leave by 10 p.m.; quiet time 10 p.m.–7 a.m.; bring your own firewood or charcoal; park store has limited supplies, snacks, drinks; pick up main supplies in Daingerfield; gathering firewood prohibited

47–52 backing up to heavy woods. The sites are large and allow a little extra privacy as you get farther from the road. Although they may not show on the park map, the interior area of Cedar Ridge includes sites 53–58, which can't be reserved ahead of time but are for tent campers and assigned by the park staff upon arrival.

Leaving this area, the restrooms and showers are directly across the road. To the right is Mountain View Camping Area, which has RVs but also a family-friendly atmosphere. To the left, you return to the day-use area and beautiful views of Lake Daingerfield, without the roar of jet boats or jet skis to interrupt your visit and enjoyment of this deep Northeast Texas park.

While this park may not be well known outside East Texas, it is very popular, so make your reservations early. The 80-acre lake was formed by an earthen dam, which was built by the CCC at the same time as the stone Boat House. There is a large swimming platform—a reminder that the local swimming hole for many generations was not a cement structure in somebody's backyard. As in days of old, meet your camping neighbors at the Pavilion on Saturday nights for music from a recently added jukebox and Dancing Under the Stars.

Camping at this low-key, low-stress park provides the perfect time to read a good book or just sit under a shade tree and reflect upon where modern civilization has taken us and what it has taken away from us.

VOICES FROM THE CAMPFIRE AND RECOMMENDED READING

The fear of death follows from the fear of life. A man who lives fully is prepared to die at any time. . . . Love implies anger. The man who is angered by nothing cares about nothing.
Edward Abbey, *A Voice Crying in the Wilderness* (New York, St. Martin's Press, 1989).

Only those are fit to live who do not fear to die; and none are fit to die who have shrunk from the joy of life and the duty of life. Both life and death are parts of the same Great Adventure.
Theodore Roosevelt, The Great Adventure (New York, Charles Scribner's Sons, 1918).

BACKCOUNTRY ADVENTURES

While the 2.5-mile hiking trail or a rental canoe, kayak, paddleboard, or boat might be enough for a nice afternoon, head up to Atlanta State Park for a touch of wild Texas. This lesser-known park sits on several ridgelines that will make your hike or bike trek a little more strenuous. It also sits on the huge Wright Patman Lake for all your open water sports.

BEST LOCAL FOOD AND DRINK

Daingerfield offers Fran's (903-645-2461) for lunch and dinner, and Hawkins (903-645-3966) serves good breakfast and lunch specials. In nearby Hughes Springs, check out Don Juan's (903-639-1721; donjuansmex.com) for Mexican food or JB's Pittsburg Hot Links (903-639-3127). Or stop by the Wildflower Inn (903-639-7342) for breakfast anytime or its home-cooked lunch buffet.

Daingerfield State Park

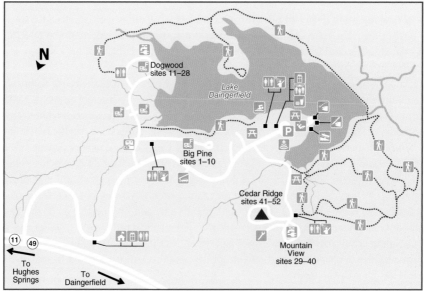

GETTING THERE

From Daingerfield, travel 3 miles east on TX 49. Park Road 17 is on the left.

GPS COORDINATES: N33° 0.750' W94° 41.466'

50

Tyler State Park

Beauty: ★★★★ / Privacy: ★★★ / Spaciousness: ★★★ / Quiet: ★★★ / Security: ★★★★ / Cleanliness: ★★★★

Tyler State Park has the feel of a more remote national park.

At one time or another, most Texans have traveled on I-20 heading for the eastern United States and those family "vacations" to see relatives or find the white sands (and mosquitos) of Florida. On those trips, most travelers have cruised at a high speed past the sign for Tyler State Park with only a quick thought as to what that park might hold. Taking the FM 14 exit and turning north for a mere 2.0 miles, the lucky tent camper will find a real surprise and a 980-acre park developed by the Civilian Conservation Corps between 1935 and 1941. These unemployed men between the ages of 17 and 25 were unwilling victims of the Great Depression and qualified for public assistance. They were paid $30 per month, of which $25 was sent home to their families. In return for backbreaking manual labor, the men received food, clothing, medical care, and tents over their heads. The state of Texas and the nation received beautiful and sturdy structures that form the foundations of many of our most beloved parks, including Tyler State Park.

As you pass the entrance station, note the Whispering Pines Nature Trail on your left, where a quiet walk will lead to many of the plants native to East Texas, including post oaks, blackjack oaks, flowering dogwoods, and redbuds. Be alert to occasional poison ivy and as with all hikes, stay on the marked trail. While enjoying the flora, also watch for the striking

East Texas camping at its best; photo credit: *Chase Fountain*

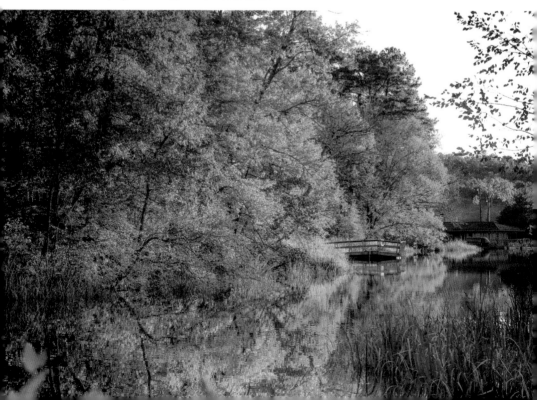

KEY INFORMATION

ADDRESS: 789 Park Road 16, Tyler, TX 75706

CONTACT: 903-597-5338, tpwd.texas.gov/state-parks/tyler

OPERATED BY: Texas Parks & Wildlife Department

OPEN: Year-round

SITES: 36 tent-only sites

EACH SITE: Picnic table, fire ring, upright charcoal grate, water

ASSIGNMENT: First come, first served until site-specific reservation system begins in 2018

REGISTRATION: At headquarters or reserve at texas.reserveworld.com or 512-389-8900

FACILITIES: Centrally located showers and modern restrooms

PARKING: At each site

FEE: $16 water-only sites; $6/person entrance fee, age 12 and under free

ELEVATION: 618'

RESTRICTIONS:

PETS: On leash only

FIRES: In fire rings or upright charcoal grates only

ALCOHOL: Prohibited in all public/outdoor areas

VEHICLES: 2/site

OTHER: Maximum 8 people/site; guests must leave by 10 p.m.; quiet time 10 p.m.–6 a.m.; bring your own firewood or charcoal; limited supplies at park store; pick up main supplies in Tyler; gathering firewood prohibited

red color of the male cardinal, the tufted titmouse, the red-bellied woodpecker, and the ever-present gray squirrel.

Returning to the trailhead, travel 0.4 mile to the Park Road 16 turnoff on your left. This narrow, paved roadway almost immediately plunges you deeper into the forest. The hilly ravine-crossed area has the look and feel of a more-remote national park such as Shenandoah or Great Smoky Mountains. The dense understory is sheltered by a 75- to 100-year-old pine-hardwood forest that acts as a time capsule of what the early pioneers to Texas would have faced as they left their worn-out lands in the east and traveled by foot, horseback, and wagon to the frontier territory of Tejas in search of new farmland or even a new life.

Go past Areas 9 and 10 (shelters) and look for Area 8/Sumac Bend campground 0.6 mile on your right. The campground road leads to sites 142–149, which run along a small, seasonal stream and are nicely spaced for privacy. Sites 146 and 149 have the feel of being deep in the woods, and the tall trees are dense enough to provide cool shade even on a hot summer visit.

Returning to the main park road, a right turn after 0.1 mile leads the tent camper to Hickory Hollow and sites 131–141. Sites 131, 132, and 134 back up to the same seasonal stream as Sumac Bend, and the sound of birds singing and squirrels racing around fill the otherwise quiet forest. Continue to sites 135–138, which border the backwater areas and are large enough for big families to spread out and enjoy the nature trail that crosses the water on a wooden bridge within a few steps of your tent site. Back on the surprisingly hilly main road, a right turn brings you to Area 6/Red Oak campground and sites 117–130. These sites are spread on an elevated ridgeline and will get a little more breeze than the lower sites. Sites 124 and 126 have partial lake views. Sites 118 and 119 are more remote and overlook a dense green canyon (OK, just a really nice ravine). Back at the turnoff, you will find the updated showers and modern restrooms on your immediate left.

Continue on for 0.2 mile to find Area 5/Dogwood Ridge Camping Area and sites 108–116. These sites are also elevated, and 111–134 have a lake view through the trees.

After you leave Area 5, the remainder of the park drive will take you to the 16 miles of bicycle trails starting at Area 4/Black Jack. Go past RV Area 3/Big Pines (no tents allowed . . . thank goodness) and finish with the lakeside sites of Area 2. While these sites must be shared with the RV crowd, the spacing is adequate and lakefront property does have its advantages.

After leaving Area 2, the bathhouse, swimming area, and Browns Point day-use area are 0.5 mile down the road. This area is very inviting on a hot day—be sure to spend a few hours swimming, fishing, or paddling around the 64-acre clear spring-fed lake. Visit the park store to rent a canoe, kayak, paddleboard, or paddleboat, and enjoy time on this peaceful lake. Whatever activity you choose, this hidden East Texas park is a gem of a forest getaway.

VOICES FROM THE CAMPFIRE AND RECOMMENDED READING

Each person has a sacred duty to use their talents to make a difference. To do otherwise is to waste the very limited time on this earth. To leave a positive legacy is a goal worth pursuing. To inspire others to leave a positive legacy is a gift to the future.
  Wendel A. Withrow, journal entry, October 16, 2004.

I never thought of myself as an environmentalist until people began to call me one. I still have trouble with the "radical environmentalist" label. It doesn't offend me; it just doesn't fit. Radicals, to me, do radical things, such as poison the water and air, eradicate hardwoods, and destroy wildlife habitat.
  Richard M. Donovan, *Paddling the Wild Neches* (College Station, Texas A&M University Press, 2006).

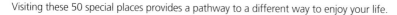

Visiting these 50 special places provides a pathway to a different way to enjoy your life.

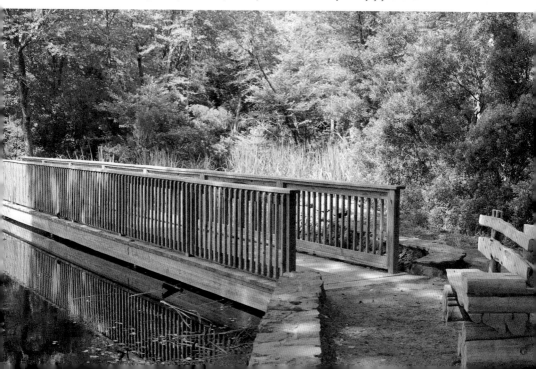

BACKCOUNTRY ADVENTURES

This beautiful and popular park has become a mecca for biking and hiking. The 16 miles of trails traverse the steep ravines, and the towering tree cover gives enough shade for a great morning ride. Be sure to bring plenty of water and snacks to be out for a few hours and just far enough away to feel the excitement of the deep forest.

BEST LOCAL FOOD AND DRINK

The ever-growing city of Tyler has plenty of good spots, including barbecue at Stanley's (903-593-0311; stanleysfamous.com) or at Bodacious (Troup Highway: 903-592-4148; Frankston Highway: 903-525-9844; thebodaciousbbq.com). For Mexican food, locals recommend Posados (Tyler: 903-405-3378; Lindale: 903-881-0434; posados.com), which has locations in Tyler and the nice town of Lindale to the east. If you're craving home cooking in Lindale, stop by Petty's Steak & Catfish (903-882-9510).

Tyler State Park

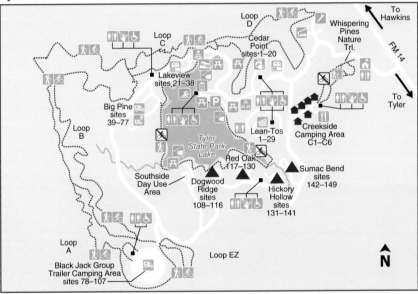

GETTING THERE

From Tyler, travel east on I-20 to the FM 14 exit. Go north on FM 14 for 2 miles. Turn left onto PR 16; park entrance is on the left.

GPS COORDINATES: N32° 28.938′ W95° 17.016′

APPENDIX A:

SOURCES OF INFORMATION

BOOKS AND MAPS

Awbrey, Betty Dooley and Stuart Awbrey. *Why Stop? A Guide to Texas Historical Roadside Markers,* 6th edition (Lanham, MD: Taylor Trade Publishing, 2013).

Big Bend Official National Park Handbook (Washington, D.C.: U.S. Department of the Interior, 1983).

Cooksey, Mel and Ron Weeks. *A Birder's Guide to the Texas Coast,* 5th edition (Delaware City: American Birding Association, 2006).

Gunter, Pete A.Y. *The Big Thicket: An Ecological Reevaluation* (Denton: University of North Texas Press, 1993).

Little, Mickey. *Hiking and Backpacking Trails of Texas,* 6th edition (Lanham, MD: Taylor Trade Publishing, 2005).

MAPSCO: The Roads of Texas (Blue Bell, PA: Kappa Map Group, 2017).

Maxwell, Ross A. *The Big Bend of the Rio Grande: A Guide to the Rocks, Landscape, Geologic History, and Settlers of the Area of Big Bend National Park* (Austin: University of Texas, 1968).

Parent, Laurence. *Hiking Big Bend National Park: A Guide to the Big Bend Area's Greatest Hiking Adventures,* 3rd edition (Guilford, CT: FalconGuides, 2015).

———. *Official Guide to Texas State Parks and Historic Sites,* revised edition (Austin: University of Texas, 2008).

Peacock, Howard. *Nature Lover's Guide to the Big Thicket* (College Station: Texas A&M University Press, 1994).

Steely, James Wright. *The Civilian Conservation Corps in Texas State Parks* (Austin: Texas Parks & Wildlife, 2010). Available as a PDF at tpwd.texas.gov/publications.

Texas Public Campgrounds: A guide to federal, state and local government administered facilities (Austin: Texas Department of Transportation, 2015). Available as a PDF at txdot.gov/inside-txdot/forms-publications/publications/travel.html.

Texas State Parks: Official Guide (Austin: Texas Parks & Wildlife, 2017). Available as a PDF at tpwd.texas.gov/state-parks/guide.

CONTACT INFORMATION

RECREATION.GOV 877-444-6777

TEXAS DEPARTMENT OF TRANSPORTATION
Travel Information Division and Office of the Governor, Economic Development, and Tourism
    txdot.gov/travel
    traveltexas.com
    800-452-9292

TEXAS PARKS & WILDLIFE tpwd.texas.gov
Reservations: tpwd.state.tx.us/reserve; 512-389-8900

US ARMY CORPS OF ENGINEERS corpslakes.us

U.S. FOREST SERVICE www.fs.fed.us

The summit at Enchanted Rock *(see page 44)*

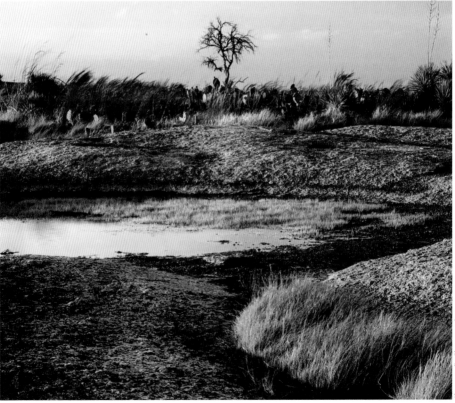

Photo credit: *Shutterstock*

APPENDIX B:

CAMPING EQUIPMENT CHECKLIST

COOKING UTENSILS

Aluminum foil
Bottle opener
Can opener
Corkscrew
Cups, plastic or tin
Dish soap (biodegradable), sponge,
    and towel
Flatware
Frying pan
Fuel for stove
Matches in waterproof container
Plates
Pocketknife
Pot with lid
Salt, pepper, spices, sugar, cooking oil,
    and maple syrup in spill-proof containers
Spatula
Stove
Wooden spoon

FIRST AID KIT

Adhesive bandages
Antibiotic cream
Blister prevention/treatment pads
Diphenhydramine (Benadryl)
Gauze pads
Ibuprofen, aspirin, acetaminophen
Insect repellent
Lip balm
Moleskin
Sunscreen
Tape, waterproof adhesive
Tweezers (to remove ticks)

SLEEPING GEAR

Pillow
Sleeping bag
Sleeping pad, inflatable or insulated
Tent with ground tarp, rainfly, extra stakes

MISCELLANEOUS

Bath soap (biodegradable), washcloth, and towel
Camp chair
Candles
Compass
Cooler
Deck of cards
Duct tape
Fire starter
Flashlight or headlamp with fresh batteries
Maps (road, topographic, trail, and so on)
Paper towels
Plastic zip-top bags
Raingear
Sunglasses
Toilet paper
Water bottle
Wool or fleece blanket

OPTIONAL

Binoculars
Field guides
Fishing rod and tackle
Grill
Hatchet
Hiking poles
Kayak and related paddling gear
Lantern
Mountain bike and related riding gear

APPENDIX C:

TOP 10 EQUIPMENT TIPS
(From Spartan to Luxury)

1. Buy a tent big enough so you don't feel claustrophobic if weather keeps you inside for a few hours but that doesn't look like a three-bedroom house (unless you brought the entire family for a week's stay).

2. Bring comfortable camp chairs for sitting around the fire.

3. Bring headlamps for tasks that require both hands to be free, a small battery-operated lamp for inside your tent (don't forget your journal or a book), and a larger lamp for lighting your cooking area or to set up your tent (turn it off as soon as your fire gets going).

4. Pack a lightweight long-sleeve shirt and pants for cool evenings or early mornings.

5. Spend the extra money to get two premium ground pads and extrawide sleeping bags. Remember, you're not backpacking, so weight and size are not a concern.

6. Bring proper-fitting hiking boots, water bottles, hats, and sun protection.

7. Bring your own dry firewood and kindling if allowed by the park. Avoid newspaper as a starter material. A small amount of solid fireplace starter or self-lighting charcoal will help in bad weather. Pack your stove on every trip in case of a burn ban or specific cooking need.

8. Slip-on camp shoes with rubber soles are a must after a long day of hiking or for walks to the bathroom. Water shoes or sandals will serve this purpose unless weather dictates otherwise.

9. Cookware should be nonstick to assist in cleanup. If you have a perfectly seasoned cast-iron skillet or Dutch oven, be sure you bring the necessary tools to clean it.

10. Food selection can be the highlight of any tent-camping experience. Fill the ice chest with goodies, but remember that this is supposed to be a vacation for everyone, including the cook and cleanup crew.

APPENDIX D:

DAY HIKING IN TEXAS

PREHIKE

Being prepared for a hike will give you the best chance of having a stress-free experience in nature. Here are a few things to consider:

1. What time of year will you be hiking?
2. Check the weather forecast a few days ahead of time and again before you leave home the day of your hike. Bring warmer clothes that you can wear in layers and raingear as indicated.
3. Pay close attention to the hike description, so you will know what preparation is necessary to have a safe and enjoyable adventure.
4. Do an equipment check at least a few days before your hike. What do you already have? What can you borrow or what do you need to buy?
5. Research any new areas for historical background or special destinations you may want to visit nearby or while driving to/from your hiking destination. (Don't forget unique food stops or shopping opportunities along the way.)
6. Plan your trail snacks/lunch ahead of time so you won't be buying at the last minute or searching your pantry for 2-year-old leftovers.
7. Always carry a day pack (small backpack) on any hike. Pack it before you start your adventure. How much does it weigh? Do you have enough water, food, clothing, and supplies to stay out on the trail for the anticipated time and longer if you're delayed?
8. Pack your daily medicines just in case you stay out longer than expected.
9. Put together a small first aid/safety kit that you can take on an everyday hike. If you're on a group hike, your leader may be required to carry a first aid kit, but you should have your own supply of the following:
   - Adhesive bandages/gauze
   - Sunscreen and sunglasses
   - Whistle (whistles carry farther than your voice)
   - Matches
   - Small knife with scissors and tweezers
   - Light source (flashlight, headlamp, or fully charged phone with light feature)
   - Watch or similar timepiece (not just cell phone)
10. Study your trail maps ahead of time, and bring them with you on every hike, along with a compass. You should know how to use both of these just in case you get separated from the group.

11. Know your physical limitations. You will have more fun, feel better, and hike farther if you get in a little better shape before you hit the trail. Take the stairs at work. Walk around the block at lunch or when you get home from work. Dust off that old treadmill in the garage. Use the exercise center at work, or at least walk past it a few times and feel healthier.

12. Chat with the park rangers before going on the trail. They're a great resource, providing suggestions and also alerting you to any changes to the trail or surroundings.

13. Know the local emergency contact number and directions to the nearest medical facility. Having a copy of this information in your pack (for while you're on the trail) and in your car will keep you from wasting time and battery life on your phone in the unlikely event that you need help. Also keep in mind that you may be in an area that doesn't get cell coverage.

GETTING READY TO HIT THE TRAIL!

1. Use a thin pair of liner socks under a medium pair of hiking socks. Synthetic material is preferred but not required. Try to stay away from cotton. This is the best defense against blisters. Remember to take these socks with you to wear if you're trying on new boots.

2. Wear light to medium hiking boots that you have already broken in walking around your neighborhood or local park. Sturdy walking shoes you already have are probably OK, but they need good tread and should be able to withstand occasional rocks and hilly terrain. Sandals, flip-flops, or slide-ons are comfy around camp but should not be worn on the trail.

3. Long pants are better so you won't have to worry about overgrown brush and the occasional poison ivy or thorns reaching out to welcome you to the wild. Lightweight hiking or fly-fishing pants are ideal, but a loose-fitting and well-worn pair of jeans will work just fine if there's no threat of rain and it's not too hot.

4. Short-sleeve shirts are great for the heat but don't give you much sun protection. Be sure to use your sunscreen or cover up with a lightweight long-sleeve shirt as necessary. Tank tops or sleeveless tops don't mix well with pack straps or the Texas sun.

5. A hat is critical. A full brim hat is the best to cover your face, ears, and neck, but a baseball cap is the minimum and will be required for summer hikes. A cap and lightweight poncho will also come in handy in case of a rainstorm.

6. Water, water, water. At least two 1-liter (32-ounce) bottles will be needed for all trips lasting 2 hours or more. Camelback or similar pouch-type hydration systems are acceptable if you know how to use them. Level indicators are strongly recommended so you can tell how much you're drinking. Consider carrying some of your water in a leak-proof container because pouch systems can sometimes leak.

7. Other than your socks and boots, your day pack is probably one of your most important items.
   - It carries your water.
   - It keeps your hands free to take pictures, carry trekking poles or a walking stick, and lend a hand to help a fellow hiker up a steep incline.
   - It carriers your food, medicine, and other essentials.
   - It needs to be sturdy enough to carry the weight, including water, which adds 2.2 pounds per liter.

- Even the cheap day packs will get you through one hike . . . maybe. Buy or borrow a better one so you can use the adjustment features. Most veteran hikers have a closet full of packs for every possible type of day hike or backpack trip. Just ask to see their secret stash, and in their enthusiasm for your getting out on the trail, they may loan you what you need.
- Packs with any kind of a hip belt and sternum strap will increase your enjoyment. The hip belts take most of the weight off your shoulders and onto your hips, providing better balance and more comfort.

8. High-tech trekking poles are helpful but not required. A sturdy wooden stick, even one found on the trail, will often work. Note: That veteran hiker friend may also have a walking stick or two . . . or ten.

9. Regarding food, just take what you like as long as it's not in a glass jar or heavy metal container. Favorite trail snacks include:
   - GORP (good ol' raisins and peanuts)
   - Trail mix from any grocery store (or make your own from items in bulk food bins at local stores such as Central Market, Sprouts, and Whole Foods)
   - Cheese and crackers (hard cheeses work better/last longer)
   - Summer sausage, cheese, crackers, and honey (mmm . . . good!)
   - Bring your own creation (sandwiches or wraps, but watch the mayo or anything else that might spoil or be messy)
   - Emergency supply of Oreo cookies, chocolate, or another favorite treat to give you that last burst of energy to get back to the trailhead.

10. Always remember safety first, especially if a thunder- or lightning storm is nearby or can be heard in the distance. Watch out for one of those famous black, blue, or green clouds that often have a Texas tornado hiding inside. Get off the trail and into a sturdy structure, or hightail it back to your car to wait it out.

11. Practice good trail etiquette.
    - If you pack it in, pack it out. Don't leave trash or uneaten foods along the trail or in the wild. This includes banana peels, orange peels, toilet   paper, or other things you believe are biodegradable.
    - Don't leave the marked trails unless necessary.
    - Don't use your cell phone on the trail unless it's an emergency.
    - Keep your voice low. Have respect for your fellow hikers and don't scare off the wildlife grazing around the next bend in the trail.

12. Don't hike alone! Make sure someone in the group knows that you are leaving the trail for a bathroom break.

13. If on a group hike, don't leave the group without your leader knowing it and making sure it can be done safely. Also, many day hikes can be broken up into shorter hikes, but doing so defeats the purpose of having a group experience. Cooperate with your leader so everyone enjoys the experience.

14. What if I see a snake or other dangerous critter? Leave it alone! It's no happier to see you than you are to see it. Back up and wait or take a safe shortcut around it.

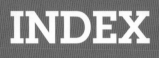

INDEX

ABOUT THE AUTHOR

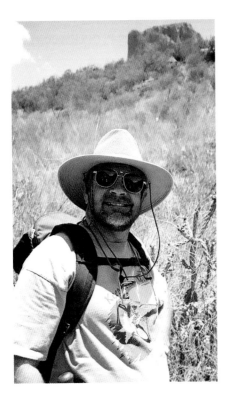

Wendel Withrow is a native Texan who began treks into the woods at a young age. During his years at the University of Texas at Austin, where he received his BA in history with high honors, Wendel began his camping career and developed a wanderlust that has taken him to the most remote and beautiful parts of Texas. After receiving his law degree from the Texas Tech University School of Law, he continued to search out the lesser-known natural wonders and historic landmarks throughout Texas and the United States. In 1989 he stumbled on *Desert Solitaire* by Edward Abbey, and his love for the outdoors was transformed into a crusade to try and save all things wild while any remained to be saved. Joining the Sierra Club, Wendel used his passion for photography and inspiration from Abbey to rise to the chair of the Lone Star Chapter and the Dallas group of the Sierra Club. Wendel continues to seek adventure in the outdoors and is currently planning educational field trips to help others experience the unique heritage and wilderness we all share as Texans.

Most recently, the Memnosyne Institute named Wendel as the director of Green Source DFW, an all-digital environmental newspaper and community resource seeking to inspire and coordinate the ever-growing number of local green-minded groups and their dedicated supporters. Finally, just in case any hours remain in the week, he is the founder of ExplorersAcademyUSA.org, a nonprofit organization dedicated to bringing outdoor adventure and appreciation to all ages and groups previously denied the opportunities many of us take for granted.

You can access photos and additional information and leave comments or ask questions at menasharidge.com/wendel or wendel@withrowlaw.com.

DEAR CUSTOMERS AND FRIENDS,

SUPPORTING YOUR INTEREST IN OUTDOOR ADVENTURE, travel, and an active lifestyle is central to our operations, from the authors we choose to the locations we detail to the way we design our books. Menasha Ridge Press was incorporated in 1982 by a group of veteran outdoorsmen and professional outfitters. For many years now, we've specialized in creating books that benefit the outdoors enthusiast.

Almost immediately, Menasha Ridge Press earned a reputation for revolutionizing outdoors- and travel-guidebook publishing. For such activities as canoeing, kayaking, hiking, backpacking, and mountain biking, we established new standards of quality that transformed the whole genre, resulting in outdoor-recreation guides of great sophistication and solid content. Menasha Ridge Press continues to be outdoor publishing's greatest innovator.

The folks at Menasha Ridge Press are as at home on a whitewater river or mountain trail as they are editing a manuscript. The books we build for you are the best they can be, because we're responding to your needs. Plus, we use and depend on them ourselves.

We look forward to seeing you on the river or the trail. If you'd like to contact us directly, visit us at menasharidge.com. We thank you for your interest in our books and the natural world around us all.

SAFE TRAVELS,

Bob Sehlinger

BOB SEHLINGER
PUBLISHER